BREAST CANCER JOURNAL

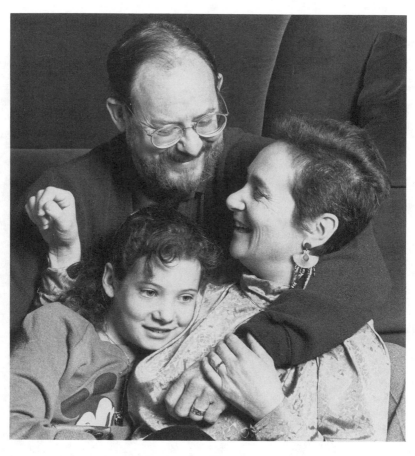

The author with her family shortly after chemotherapy ended.
Photo courtesy of Laura Rauch.

B R E A S T
C A N C E R
J O U R N A L

a century of petals

JULIET WITTMAN

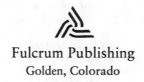

Fulcrum Publishing
Golden, Colorado

First Fulcrum trade paperback edition published October 1994.

The author would like to thank the following for permission to reprint:

Excerpt from *You're Only Old Once!* by Dr. Seuss. Copyright © 1986 by Theodor S. Geisel and Audrey S. Geisel, Trustees under Trust Agreement dated August 27, 1984. Reprinted by permission of Random House, Inc.

Excerpt from *The Lady's Not for Burning* © 1950. Renewed 1978 by Christopher Fry. Quoted by permission of Flora Roberts, Inc.

Library of Congress Cataloging-in-Publication Data

Wittman, Juliet.
    Breast cancer journal : a century of petals / Juliet Wittman.
        p.   cm.
    Includes bibliographical references.
    ISBN 1-55591-136-6
    ISBN 1-55591-194-3 (pbk.)
    1. Wittman, Juliet—Health.   2. Breast—Cancer—Patients—United States—Biography.   3. Breast—Cancer.   4. Breast—Cancer—Information services.   I. Title.
RC280.B8W53   1993
362.1'9699449'092—dc20
[B]   92-54765
                                                        CIP

Printed in the United States of America
0 9 8 7 6 5 4 3 2 1

Fulcrum Publishing
350 Indiana Street, Suite 350
Golden, CO 80401–5093
(800) 992-2908

For my parents:

Gabriella Erdelyi
Edward Erdelyi
Desider Robert Wittman

CONTENTS

FOREWORD
By Paul K. Hamilton, M.D.

I accepted the author's invitation to read the manuscript and write the foreword with some ambivalence, as I have a number of bestsellers totally or partially unread on my bedside table. However, once I started reading the manuscript, I found that, after the first few pages, I was captivated by the author's creative writing and the authenticity of her work.

Breast Cancer Journal is a story of a young woman's search for tools to cope with cancer and the surgery and chemotherapy that ensued after her diagnosis. Despite the progress in cancer treatment, most people still equate the word with death. The fear of mutilating surgery, the fear of pain, and the fear of the side effects of treatment are often overwhelming and lead to feelings of a loss of control of one's life and destiny. The author chronicles these emotions in a most poignant way. She tells how her creativity and daring to be vulnerable lead her to persons who support her and bond with her, promoting a healing of her spirit. She describes how she was able to get in touch with her own "inner healer" and find love and acceptance.

In 1986, with a few patients and health professionals, I founded the QuaLife Wellness Community. I am very grateful that the author participated in the Pathways to Healing weekend of QuaLife, which she describes in this book. She experienced the power and healing of a caring and compassionate community composed of patients, their significant others and health professionals.

I am confident that this book will be of immense help to women who have breast cancer and who are searching themselves for empowerment, courage and hope. Indeed, anyone facing a life-challenging illness will find the book instructive and supportive. I believe that, from reading it, family members will gain a clearer understanding of the turbulent journey their loved ones undertake when they face cancer. All health professionals, especially oncologists, surgeons and oncology nurses, will benefit immensely by taking this journey with the author.

I plan to obtain copies of *Breast Cancer Journal* to distribute to patients I encounter in my practice and to those I meet at QuaLife. It is a remarkable and loving journal of a spirit journey.

ACKNOWLEDGMENTS

I hope the friends who lent their loving support, and the doctors, nurses and technicians who so skillfully took care of me will consider themselves sufficiently thanked in the pages that follow. There are a few others, however, to whom my debt of gratitude is also great:

John Thorndike, Claudia Putnam, Pat Wagenhals, Ellen Zweibel and Tim Hillmer for their comments and criticisms on this manuscript.

Caryn McVoy for our working weekends at the Foot of the Mountain Motel and our long nourishing talks about writing.

Meg Ruley of the Jane Rotrosen Agency, whose faith in this book enabled me to finish it.

Alix Kates Shulman for her encouragement and support.

Judy Anderson who taught me to see, who can make dreams and ideas visible and who did the cover illustration for this book.

Fulcrum Publishing, in particular Bob Baron (tallest publisher in the West), Linda Stark, Sandra Trupp and Carmel Huestis for her thoughtful and sensitive editing.

Barbara Demaree, Becky Jancosko, Ana Claire and Peter Davison of Ballet Arts, who provided spiritual sustenance, a place of refuge and excellent technical training for my daughter during some of the hardest months of her life.

And Bill; and Anna, who is my heart.

*... I can pass to you
Generations of roses in this wrinkled berry.
There: now you hold in your hand a race
Of summer gardens, it lies under centuries
Of petals. What is not, you have in your palm.
Rest in the riddle, rest.*

—Christopher Fry, *The Lady's Not for Burning*

BREAST CANCER JOURNAL

1
DIAGNOSIS

May 1988. It was my doctor on the phone. He was talking gravely about the results of my mammogram. "There are clusters of calcification," he said, and I breathed a quick sigh of relief—he hadn't used the word *cancer*—but then he went on. "Abnormal. The radiologist is adamant the lump should be biopsied."

I waited for some word of reassurance, some platitude about most breast lumps not being cancer, some nonthreatening medical explanation for the soft knot in my breast. Reassurance generally came easily to this courtly gentleman of a doctor, who had delivered my daughter ten years ago and taken care of my gynecological needs ever since. His silence was threatening. I said, "Dr. Spencer, I'm afraid."

He sounded almost irritated. "Well, I did suggest a mammogram," he said, as if I'd tried to deny it. Then he went on. "I've made an appointment for you to consult with a surgeon at the Boulder Medical Center at three o'clock. His name's Dr. Day. He'll be doing the biopsy. He's very good."

Soon after this conversation, a friend, Diana Somerville, arrived at the newspaper where I worked as features editor to discuss a series of freelance articles. In the haze of fear that followed my conversation with the doctor, I'd tried to call and cancel our appointment, but there'd been no answer. Now I was glad of her presence.

We went into an empty room, and I told her what had happened. She said two of her friends had had breast cancer. A few days ago, she'd driven one of them to a doctor's appointment to get the stitches from her reconstruction removed. The other had had chemotherapy, and marijuana had helped her control the resultant nausea.

3

I was drifting through this conversation, distracted and passive. Then I was hit by a wave of panic. We were talking as if it were a foregone conclusion that I had cancer. "I don't want to have to do those things," I said. "I don't want to go through any of that." She slipped smoothly into reassurance: "And you probably won't have to."

At quarter of three, I asked my co-workers to look out for my ten-year-old daughter, Anna, who was walking over from ballet later for a ride home with me. I asked them to tell her there'd been a hitch in plans, and she was to wait: eventually I or her father would pick her up. Then Diana drove me to the medical center. We were a few minutes early, so we pulled into a small park nearby. Three children were playing ball; adults strolled in the sun; a curly black dog investigated the edge of a flowerbed. I wanted time to stop.

There are several physical manifestations of fear. Somehow, during the course of that strange afternoon, I became intimately acquainted with all of them. There's the choking sensation that threatens to cut off your breath. There's the weakness in the knees that causes you to stumble going up the stairs. And there's another feeling. The feeling that you're lost somewhere in space, turning and turning in the black ether, while slowly, very slowly and starting from the heart, your entire body turns to ice.

Dr. John Day, who found me in tears on the examining table, was a good bit younger than Dr. Spencer and seemed awkward. He palpated the lump, then had me close my robe and led me out into the corridor to show me a slide from the mammogram—a gray blur against a white wall. "I want you to look at this," he said, gently, insistently. "I want you to understand this." But I couldn't fix my attention. This was the image that had betrayed me. So he explained the fuzzy shadows in detail to my husband, Bill, who had somehow miraculously appeared in his office— summoned, I supposed, by a call from my co-workers. Or had I phoned him? I couldn't remember.

But Day's hand as he took the film down from the wall, his face, everything, came into blinding focus with his next words.

"We need to do a biopsy Thursday. I'd say from this there's a better than sixty percent chance you have cancer."

In the two days between those words and the biopsy, I never really doubted that I did.

Two months earlier, I'd visited with an old friend who was ill with cancer. Cecile Lazar's life and that of my family had been interwoven for years. When my parents first came to Colorado, she had befriended my mother, helping ease her loneliness. Then the two of them had conspired to ensure that Cecile's daughter, Lynn, and I met. Probably despite, rather than because of, our mothers' friendship, we became fast friends. Now Lynn, her husband, Gunner Kaersvang, and their eleven-year-old daughter, Dana, represented a kind of extended family for Bill, Anna and me.

Cecile had helped and supported me through my mother's final illness and death, and it followed naturally that, hours after I had given birth to Anna, she should appear at my hospital bed— as she had by Lynn's seven months earlier—bearing a gift of chopped chicken liver and accompanied by her husband, Joe. They had gotten past the staff by signing in as Anna's grandparents.

When I visited her, Cecile had already undergone the entire panoply of cancer treatments. Surgery had removed the lump she'd found at the side of her face, where her jawbone joined her neck. Although the surgeons believed they had removed all trace of malignancy, the lump had grown back—so fast that Cecile said she could feel the cells multiplying day by day. Radiation had followed the surgery, and several bouts with the chemotherapeutic agent doxorubicin, generally known as Adriamycin, followed that. The conjunction of radiation and chemotherapy had raised an ugly, blistering burn where the original lump had been removed.

Now the cancer was in Cecile's lungs. Still, she felt well and remained commandingly herself. The only evidence of illness was a phlegmy cough that increasingly thickened and blurred her voice as the afternoon wore on. But she was determined, nonetheless, to speak. Passover was a month away, and she didn't know, she said, if she'd be well enough to prepare the seder. Would I be willing to help Lynn with the planning and cooking if necessary? Of course I would.

That settled, she sat by me on the couch, a white-haired, heavyset woman, as solid and comfortable as a wardrobe, reading some pieces of writing she'd recently put together for a living history project. The terrible fits of coughing kept interrupting the narrative, but she insisted on reading herself rather than simply handing her essays to me. Her writing, humorous, intelligent, smoothly and swiftly written, told of a life that had, in a small way, pioneered new territory. In the forties, when American women were routinely giving birth heavily drugged, she'd read about natural childbirth and—without the aid of Lamaze classes, helpful doctors and sisterly support from the feminist movement—chosen to practice it for the births of her three children. While many of her peers had stayed at home raising their families, Cecile had become a practicing psychologist.

It was impossible to believe that this vital, strong-willed woman was dying, that in a few short weeks she would simply cease to exist, that eventually the only evidence of her sharp mind, of the idiosyncratic patterns of her life, would be the writing on these pieces of paper.

Still, there was a quietness to the afternoon, a sense of—not acceptance exactly, but a kind of resignation, gentle, tinged faintly with bitterness. Earlier, Cecile—so known in our circle of friends for sudden, wounding remarks that my husband had coined the term *Cecilian slip* to describe her verbal sorties—had been terrified and angry. To offer sympathy, affection, a small gift was to invite that critical tongue into swift action against oneself. Now she was calm and kindly.

I left intending to visit again, as frequently as possible. But the next week I had flu (all sniffles and sore throats were kept far from Cecile, whose immune system had been weakened by chemotherapy), and by the week after, she was incoherent and unlikely to recognize me, Lynn said. When I visited her house again, it was to view her body. She was buried next to my parents.

6

It was a week after Cecile's funeral, a Sunday morning. I sat in our sunny living room, sipping coffee, reading the newspaper. My left hand played idly with the collar of my robe. Suddenly I stopped. Inadvertently, I had touched the place where my right breast begins to swell into fullness. And there beneath my fingers was a lump. An indisputable lump. It was as if this fleshy thickening had wanted my attention, had deliberately, insistently, pushed itself up against my fingers.

For a moment, nothing. No reaction. No fear. Just a cessation of thought and feeling, a silence as absolute as the silence that surrounds a corpse, as deep as the silence that had emanated from Cecile in the weeping house. Cecile lying on the bed, her hand grown stiff and cold, the mottled burn at the side of her face hardened into marble.

Eventually, of course, I investigated the lump. It wasn't particularly hard. When I raised my arm, changing the contour of the breast, it seemed almost to vanish, although I could feel hard little granulations beneath the place where it had been, right up against the wall of my chest. All morning, I probed—in the shower, on the bed. Sometimes, for a brief, hopeful second, I lost track of the lump altogether. Sometimes when I located it again, it was with an odd sense of relief: "Oh, there you are. And you're such an ordinary thing. Not anything so dramatic or so alien, really."

Because the lump was at once unlike anything I had ever felt and oddly familiar. It was just a kind of exaggeration of the bump caused by a large lymph node or the swell of an infected gland— little knobs and protuberances I'd encountered before. Surely it couldn't represent a serious threat.

And reason rushed to my aid. In the interior dialogue that we routinely conduct, I comforted myself with a full array of rationalizations. The lump was normal, just something that I'd never noticed before. It was connected with my menstrual cycle and would vanish later in the month. Like millions of other women, I had a fibrocystic hardening. Even: I was so upset by Cecile's death, which brought back memories of my mother's painful struggle with cancer, that I'd somehow willed this lump into being. "Just like me," I grumbled to myself, "to come up with a hysterical lump."

For a couple of weeks, I pushed all thought of the intrusion in my breast firmly back into the recesses of my mind. Then one morning, in the bath, I felt it again. This time I knew. Something was wrong. No matter how I investigated, raising and lowering my arm, circling with the pads of my fingers, checking the left breast to see if any similar thickening existed there, I couldn't make the lump go away. And I finally acknowledged that it was unlike anything I'd ever felt in my breast before. I called the Boulder Medical Center and made an appointment with Dr. Spencer. I also asked for a mammogram.

Then I broke down. It seemed unfair to burden Lynn so soon after the death of her mother, and something in me wanted to keep my stark panic from my husband. So I called another friend, Caryn McVoy, and poured out my fears. My mother had died of cancer, I told her, and so had my father—at the age of forty-six. My forty-sixth birthday was days away. Was I destined to follow my father?

I must have been babbling. I talked about a business conference I was supposed to attend in Philadelphia at the end of the week, and how I was now afraid to go, afraid the plane would crash, afraid to be away from Bill and Anna.

Cecile's entire odyssey had begun with a little lump at the side of her face.

Swiftly, lovingly, Caryn came to my rescue. She talked about breast lumps and how common they were. Almost all of them turned out to be fibrocystic, she said. She herself had often found lumps: "They feel sort of like peeled grapes."

"Yes, yes," I concurred eagerly. "That's exactly how it feels."

In the course of the next week I would discover that almost all women share a mythology of breast cancer. It's as if a stream of ideas and images circling this topic moves continuously from woman to woman. We lean toward each other, share information in low, confiding voices. "It happened to me once. The doctor said we should watch it." Or, "I'm always lumpy. I should probably stop drinking coffee." There are questions: Is the lump very hard? Can you move it with your fingers? Where is it in your breast? Questions, observations, intimacies, everything rushes toward a final, deeply drawn breath of relief. "Oh, in that case—because it's hard, soft, movable, immovable, in the inner quadrant, out toward your armpit—it can't be cancer."

Meanwhile, on the phone, Caryn, who works as a therapist, was telling me how common it is for adults to become fearful of death when they reach the age at which a parent died.

Two days later I showed the lump to Dr. Spencer, studied his face as he examined it. It was about time for a mammogram, he said, and I should schedule one. I told him I had. Good, he responded. Not that he thought the lump was anything to worry about. It felt fibrocystic. "You've no idea," he told me, as I laughed aloud in relief, "how very hard a cancer usually feels." As he was leaving the room, he turned to me. "I wouldn't lose any sleep over this."

"I told you so," said my husband exultantly that evening. "I told you it was nothing to worry about." I relaxed for the first time that week.

But by the time I went to the medical center for the mammogram the next morning, I was afraid again. I had been running the risk factors for breast cancer over and over in my mind through the night. I had had my first child late. Bad. But perhaps a little better than never having had a child at all. I had nursed Anna for a long time. Good. Perhaps. My first menstruation had been neither particularly early nor particularly late. Late would have been best. I was perhaps a smidgen overweight—and the weight was concentrated in my midsection rather than on my buttocks or thighs. Bad. Were my breasts particularly dense—another negative? I had no idea.

There was no breast cancer that I was aware of in my family, but few of my relatives, Jews in Central Europe, had been given the chance to die of disease. Both my parents had had cancers of other kinds. I wasn't aware then that the colon cancer that had killed my mother may have had some relationship to breast cancer: a murky connection researchers sense, but no one quite understands.

At the center, a nurse asked why I'd come in, and I told her about the lump. "Well," I amended hastily, afraid that somehow naming the thing would make it real, "it wasn't exactly a lump. Sort of a ... uh ... thickening. Dr. Spencer doesn't think it's anything."

The technician who tightened the plates of the machine on my breasts was young and skinny. She was nice enough, but I wanted a middle-aged Jewish mother, with a big, soft bosom, someone who'd bullied and coaxed several children through adolescence, and who would both acknowledge and make light of my fears.

The technician asked me to wait while she checked the photos, then returned to reshoot one of them. I was terrified. I thought it meant she'd seen something wrong and wanted to get a closer look at it. I examined her closed, cool little face but found no hint there of my fate.

Later, I had lunch with a writer friend. I told her about the mammogram, hoping for the same kind of reassurances I'd heard from Caryn. Instead she said, "Breast cancer is very common. They say one woman in ten will get it. That means ... ," and she gestured toward the other people in the cozy dining room of the little Creole restaurant where we sat, "... around three of the women in this room."

Months later, I would remind her of that conversation. "Yes," she said, "but I didn't mean us. I didn't think you had cancer. I didn't think it would happen to me or you."

We walked out onto the street. The wind was coming up, the bright day turning cooler. I pulled my sweater closed around my body, but I couldn't stop the shivering.

The evening after my visit with Dr. Day, I received two phone calls. They were from the women Diana had described to me at the office that afternoon.

Leanne Barrett was a science writer I had met many years earlier, though we had not been in contact since. Her breast cancer had been diagnosed eight years ago, and she seemed living proof that the disease could be survived. But what she said disturbed me profoundly. She had had a mastectomy in Boulder, she said. Then she had gone to the M.D. Anderson Cancer Research Center in Texas, where, because the form of cancer she had was particularly virulent and likely to recur, she'd had a second mastectomy and been given a prescription for chemotherapy. Boulder doctors, said Leanne, simply weren't in touch with the latest research and were frequently unwilling to recommend the draconian remedies necessary. My life could depend on the depth and sophistication of my doctor's knowledge. In addition, surgeons who performed breast surgery at M.D. Anderson did no other kind of work and hence developed tremendous skill. In Boulder, one might be operated on by a general surgeon, who'd just come from a gall bladder operation or an appendectomy.

Ironically, it was my own stepfather, with whom she'd had some professional dealings, who had persuaded Leanne to seek treatment outside Boulder. He had always been convinced that my mother's death was due, at least in part, to the incompetence of her doctors. A short, excitable man of passionate beliefs and iron will, he'd burst into Leanne's hospital room shortly after her surgery, gesticulating and shouting at her in his heavily Hungarian-accented English that her only chance of survival was to go to a major national center for cancer research. She'd listened to him, and she was convinced that his advice had saved her life. Now he was no longer living, and she felt it was her duty to pass it on to me.

"After my surgery," she said, "I met ten breast cancer patients through the Reach for Recovery program. They all had Boulder doctors, and they all loved their doctors. That was eight years ago. Every one of them is dead now."

An hour or two later, Doris Olsen called. She, too, urged me to go to M.D. Anderson. True, she explained, the first visit there was frightening. It was a huge, impersonal facility where you could wait up to four hours to see your doctor, and where you were constantly confronted with the sight of suffering and dying people. But the doctors were kind, once reached, and the care skilled and expert.

Doris also made two more suggestions. She recommended a surgeon, Susan Darcy, for a second opinion, describing Darcy as kind, efficient and very honest. And she told me about a psychiatrist she'd visited at the height of her own panic and confusion, Antonio Wood. He'd helped her a great deal, she said. Perhaps he could help me, too.

"Dr. Day's given me Valium," I told her. "I've never taken it before, and I'm kind of afraid to take it now. I'm afraid there might be so much worse to come. ... I mean, if I have to have a mastectomy and everything. ..."

"What you're going through right now is the worst," said Doris firmly. "Nothing that comes later is as bad as the first few days, when you don't know if you have cancer or not. So do what you have to do. And take your Valium."

Coming from Doris—who'd had a double mastectomy and should know—I found this observation deeply comforting. "This is the worst," I'd tell myself, stumbling through the hours that followed, "and I'm still here. I'm still functioning."

Two days later, mammogram in hand (I was almost afraid to hold it or look at it; it seemed to make my sickness real), I visited Dr. Darcy with Bill. She examined me with cool fingers, slowly and thoroughly. Then she peered at the mammogram. "Well," she said, "I guess my estimate is a little different from Dr. Day's. A little lower. I'd say there's only a fifty percent chance you have cancer."

I was soon to find that statistics are a huge part of the cancer patient's world. There are the glib, half accurate assertions of news stories—"One woman in ten, nationwide, develops breast cancer; forty-four thousand die of the disease every year" is how almost every article on the topic begins—the educated guesses of doctors, the figures tossed around in studies and popularizations of studies. These numbers blurred and shifted constantly. I'd hear a doctor say that women whose cancers have not spread to the lymph nodes have a 90 percent chance of a normal lifespan, then read a newspaper article on whether or not these women should have chemotherapy that cited a 30 percent mortality rate. And I'd study these fluid, changing numbers frantically for a clue as to whether I was going to live or die.

In a sense, of course, all statistics are meaningless. It's irrelevant that only one in several million people will be killed by a toppled flowerpot if the flowerpot falls on you. The odds against you have just become 100 percent. Or, as my oncologist would explain to me later, "If you survive, you survive. If you die, you die. You don't end up seventy percent alive—or alive up to here ...," indicating an area roughly in the middle of his chest, "... and dead from there on up."

In the meantime, Susan Darcy added one more statistic: "Of all the women diagnosed as having breast cancer, fifty percent are dead within ten years."

The biopsy was scheduled for a Thursday at 11 A.M. At 10 A.M. I found myself in the office of the second doctor Doris had recommended—the psychiatrist Antonio Wood. This was a spacious, multi-windowed room facing directly onto a brook. Clearly, someone had paid attention to every detail here: the placement of the furniture, the arrangement of dried flowers in a deep blue vase by the door. The room emanated a sense of order and calm.

Dr. Wood himself was a slight man, with dark hair, a droll, intelligent face, an easy, responsive way of laughing. I told him I didn't want to go for the biopsy. I wanted to crawl under his desk and shelter there. I wanted to curl up in his coat pocket and have him carry me away to wherever he was going next—anywhere but the Boulder Medical Center and my impending tryst with the surgeon. How, I asked him, was I going to cover the distance from his office to the center without going mad with fear and anticipation?

I don't remember exactly what he said, but the gist of it was this: I should focus on all the sensory details I encountered on the journey. The slant of sunlight on the sidewalk, the fresh, pretty colors of the women's summer dresses, the scent of the sprig of lilac I'd brought with me from the garden as a talisman.

This advice got me there. At the center, they had me put on a gown. A nurse took the lilac and placed it in a water glass where I could see it. Then a doctor I hadn't encountered before began inserting a wire marker into my breast to show the location of the lump. This didn't hurt, because they had numbed the area, though it did seem strange to look down and see my breast bleeding. I wanted to protect it. Until that moment, the strongest emotion I'd ever associated with this right breast was connected with the memory of my newborn daughter putting her lips to it and the sweet, strong pull as she suckled.

This new doctor was very kind. Nine times out of ten, he told me, the lumps excised during biopsies are not cancerous. I was probably going to be just fine. I didn't mention Dr. Day's estimate. Or Susan Darcy's.

Just before the biopsy, a drug was injected into my veins. It seemed to rush straight to my teeming brain and clear it. Suddenly I was cheerful, unafraid. "Couldn't you keep me on this for a month or two?" I asked the nurse, and she laughed.

A green sheet prevented me from seeing what Dr. Day was doing. The nurse talked to me, held my hand, sometimes put her palms to the sides of my face through the procedure. Though I could feel a fumbling and tugging at my breast, there was no pain.

But it was a cancer. I don't remember if Dr. Day said it aloud, or if it was simply that his breathing changed, or his kidding with the nurses suddenly stopped. I just knew. And at the time, under the influence of that wondrous drug, I didn't much care.

Dr. Day was stitching me up, and one of the nurses was urging him to repeat a joke he'd told her earlier. He demurred. I thought his reluctance was because of the cancer and appreciated it, but he didn't have to refrain from joke-telling on my behalf. I wouldn't have minded. In fact, a joke suddenly seemed to me just the thing. Normal. Helpful. Finally, he told it. It was something about a gorilla.

Two hours later, in Dr. Day's office, the conversation was more serious. He'd excised a one-and-a-half-centimeter tumor. He wouldn't know until he'd talked to the lab whether to recommend a mastectomy (and what kind of mastectomy) or to be content with the lumpectomy he'd just performed. I hadn't realized before that the biopsy served as the lumpectomy.

The nurse had already shown me a booklet that explained the different kinds of mastectomy, complete with antiseptic little diagrams. It all sounded so matter-of-fact. The procedure described in the booklet had nothing to do with severing a body part, with cutting my warm, familiar breast from my body, turning it into something bloody and alien and disposing of it ... how? In some kind of refuse heap of human parts? My imagination faltered and stopped.

In any event, Day explained, even if I didn't require a mastectomy, there'd be further surgery. He needed to take the lymph nodes from under my arm and examine them. In the booklet, the lymph nodes looked like tiny grapes on a sprig. Day said he'd take as many as he could find, and for a fevered moment, I imagined him searching blindly through the bloody recesses of my armpit. But then he explained that he would just remove a lemon-sized chunk of flesh (like someone scooping a brown spot from a pear, I thought), and the lab would extract the lymph nodes from that. For the moment, he wanted me to have a chest X-ray and a blood test. I couldn't bring myself to examine the reasons. I simply went from place to place in the building, numb, complying with his orders. As a young, dark-haired technician took my blood, I told her, "I have cancer," testing the phrase. She looked distressed and sympathetic.

Later, I ran into the avuncular doctor who'd inserted the wire before the biopsy. "It was cancer," I told him, studying his face. Immediately, I saw there the same concerned expression the technician had worn.

I realized it was definite then.

I did have cancer.

15

2
SURGERY

Two days after the biopsy, Bill called Dr. Day's office because I was afraid to. He talked to Candis Cooke, the nurse. There was a margin of clear tissue around the tumor Day had excised, she said. My lungs appeared to be uninvolved. There was no evidence of spread. Still holding the receiver, Bill called the glad news out to me from our study, and I rushed in to take it from his hand. Patiently, Candis repeated her news. I had barely got the phone back in its cradle before I sank to the floor, crying in pure joy and relief.

Puzzled and afraid, Anna came into the room. "It's all right," I told her, and Bill added, "Mommy's going to be OK."

Later that evening, as I lay in bed reading, Bill sat down next to me and took my hand. "I feel as if we've been in free fall all week," he said. "I know we're not completely out of danger yet, but it feels as if our feet have at least touched the ground."

In my mind I saw a hiking boot, firmly planted on a mountain ledge. We held each other for a long time.

Anna appeared to be profoundly reassured. "I'm psychic," she told me a few days later. "I knew it was a cancer. But I knew it was going to be OK, too. It's just like with grandma Cecile. I knew she was going to die. ... " I was watching her closely, fascinated at the way she was dealing with this, half believing that she could foresee my future. "And I knew," she went on jubilantly, "that you were going to ... " She stopped. Her eyes slid away from mine. I think the intensity of my gaze unnerved her. Or she was afraid to make a prediction for fear her presumption might tempt the gods. At any rate, she couldn't say the word "live."

As her face closed to me, I ached with pity. My child was in pain, and—for what seemed like the first time—I couldn't comfort her. Now it was I who turned away.

Perhaps fortunately, this week before my surgery was a very busy time for Anna. She had a small role in a production of the ballet *Coppelia* and was in rehearsal every evening. This kept her distracted, and it was a relief for me, too. I was submerged in a kind of sea of fear and confusion, unable to help her, unwilling to let her see my condition.

I thought about dying. I dwelt obsessively on my mother's four-year struggle—from the tiny lump in her colon that the doctor hoped was a polyp, through the colostomy, the endless recurrences, the spread, the tortuous dying. That experience was etched on my brain. And on some level I believed it was the inevitable way of the disease. Intellectually I understood that there were women who survived breast cancer by five, ten, even forty years. But I knew there were others who died within a year of diagnosis. Which was I?

In his office, Dr. Day had said that when breast cancer spreads, or metastasizes, it most commonly affects the liver, the lungs, the bones or the brain.

Lying awake in the gray hours of the morning, I heard a hissing little voice, insinuating, familiar, from the depths of my own being. And what it was saying, over and over again, was simply, "Metastasis. Metastasisss."

Over the next few weeks it returned periodically, like a nightmare, until the day I confronted it. "You're nothing," I told this sinister, deathly presence. "Nothing at all. That's only a word."

On Monday I returned to work. I was taking Valium for the first time in my life, to take the edge off the fear. Dr. Wood had suggested that it was important to set up and maintain a schedule, to do whatever work I had to do meticulously and with total concentration. Accordingly, I had planted a few marigolds around the muddy vegetable garden over the weekend. Now I struggled to edit articles, return phone calls, open and sort the mail. In the midst of all this, Dr. Day called. He'd been thinking, he said, and he'd decided that I did not need a mastectomy. The biopsy-lumpectomy he had already performed would suffice. Of course,

17

he reminded me, I'd still have to undergo the lymph node dissection.

It sounded too good to be true. "Are you sure?" I asked him. "Is this the decision you'd make if I were your wife?"

He hesitated. "That's a hard one. It does mean we'll have to watch very carefully to make sure there's no recurrence. And the scar tissue will make your future mammograms more difficult to read. But, yes, the tumor was small enough, and I think we can save the breast."

Now began a mad scramble for information. By training, profession and inclination, I am a grubber after facts; the simple accumulation of data has always delighted me. And maybe, I thought, this represented a way out of the formless void where I floated, a means of finding some inner strength for the coming battles. I'd been an investigative journalist. Now I'd work on the investigation that might save my life. Ronda Haskins, the editor of the science and health section at the newspaper, gave me a folder full of articles about breast cancer. I took it home and placed it by my armchair in the living room. For two days I flirted with it, plunging into the clippings and then withdrawing, the way you edge your tongue toward an aching tooth and wince at the pain it elicits.

Finally, I sat down one night, sorted the articles into various topics and pulled out all of them that related to surgery for breast cancer. For almost a hundred years, it seemed, American doctors had routinely performed what was called a Halsted radical mastectomy on breast cancer patients. This involved not only cutting off the breast, but removing the underlying muscles and the lymph nodes and fatty tissue in the armpit—and sometimes the internal mammary nodes under the sternum as well. The patient never regained full use of her arm. I remembered, as I read, a woman I'd known when I was a child in London, a violinist who'd had a radical mastectomy in her forties. She was now in her eighties and very much alive. But she had never played the violin again.

In Europe, doctors began experimenting with less mutilating surgeries early in the century, and in the 1970s Dr. George Crile began questioning the routine use of the Halsted radical in the United States. Eventually, many women were given a choice in the matter of surgery, and even lumpectomy, which removes only the tumor and a margin of tissue around it, became relatively common.

This was good news, of course, but not entirely so. There was a reason that less draconian surgeries were becoming more acceptable. The medical establishment was learning that breast cancer is a systemic disease. While it was generally believed that there was a simple, linear progression of tumor cells from the breast to the lymph nodes and then out into the body, it made sense to take out as much tissue as possible. If the cancer recurred, the reasoning went, it was because the surgeon had not removed all traces of it. Now it was understood that by the time this slippery illness had manifested itself in a woman's breast, cancerous cells might have been disseminated throughout her body by unknown pathways as well as in the bloodstream. The focus began to shift from surgery as the primary cure to surgery as one weapon in an arsenal that included radiation and chemotherapy.

I scanned the newspaper articles for any sign of a backlash. I found there was no indication that women who had lumpectomies relapsed any more frequently than did their mastectomized sisters.

If this was true, why had so many of the women I'd met in the past couple of weeks had mastectomies, even double mastectomies? In some cases, I recalled, more extensive surgery was called for because the cancer appeared in several places in the breast, or was particularly likely to recur. The size and location of the tumor and the size and shape of the breast were also relevant. But I found out later that the decision also depended a great deal on the belief systems of both patients and doctors.

After lumpectomy, cancer recurs in the same breast 28 percent of the time—6 percent if the breast has been irradiated. It appears in the previously unaffected breast at a rate of 1 percent a year. Scar tissue from a lumpectomy can make detection of a recurrence difficult. And some doctors, who have seen patients die because a recurrence went unnoticed too long, feel that mastectomy—even double mastectomy—is safer. There are doctors who feel passionate about this, who believe that a kind of softness and misplaced pity in the profession is ultimately dooming women. There are doctors who take the same kind of hard line on chemotherapy, too, saying that harsher drugs at higher doses bring better results than the more limited protocols most practitioners are willing to prescribe.

In addition, if I had only a lumpectomy, I would have to have radiation to the breast. This was a lengthy, tiring process that carried dangers of its own.

Mastectomy? Lumpectomy? I swayed between the two options, trying to apply all the life knowledge I'd accumulated to the decision, realizing how irrelevant the bits of wisdom and understanding gleaned in other areas seemed in the face of cancer.

I realized that, to a large extent, how you visualized your cancer, the metaphor you used for it, determined the treatment you'd accept and the way you'd live with the disease. There was the concept that a single cancerous cell, anywhere in the body, would eventually kill you—which meant that if even one such cell had slipped by Dr. Day's knife during the biopsy, I was doomed. But some experts say that our bodies deal routinely with hundreds of cancerous cells, that our immune systems can protect us and that the key is keeping everything in balance.

Perhaps gardening was an appropriate metaphor. When I first became a gardener, I remembered, I'd panicked at the sight of an aphid or a squash bug, imagining the garden and my strong green seedlings devastated overnight. Yet over the years I'd learned that a few pests were necessary. They kept their own natural predators in the area. A hole nibbled in a tomato or a worm nestled in the tip of an ear of corn: these were simply part of the natural process, not harbingers of utter destruction. There were so many factors— the quality of the soil, the viability of the seed, the proportion of rain to wind and sun, the sturdiness of the seedlings, the proximity of garlic, marigolds, nasturtiums and other natural repellents— that determined whether the appearance of a single Mexican bean beetle was simply a nuisance or an indication that the entire bean crop was doomed.

So it seemed that the way to combat disease was to keep your body strong, your environment healthy. But—to take the analogy further—there was a level of attack that a garden simply could not withstand. I thought of the summer when Boulder was visited by a plague of grasshoppers. Within a week the flourishing potato vines had been eaten to the ground. Walking over the barren soil, I couldn't even tell where I had planted the potatoes. I supposed there must be cancers as voracious and unstoppable as that.

On a metaphorical level, the harshest remedies for cancer— double mastectomy, chemotherapies so potent that they some- times killed the patient—seemed the equivalent of saturating a vegetable plot with pesticide. In a grasshopper year there may be no alternative. But, as any farmer knows, a few pests always survive these onslaughts to breed next year's attacking army.

And yet. And yet. How apt was the metaphor? How valid was my sense of how things worked? My entire belief system had been blown to bits by the diagnosis of cancer.

Many months later, I discussed all this with another breast cancer patient. "Oh, yes," she said, "selecting the treatment is the most agonizing part of the entire process. Women should be told that. Your survival hinges on making the right choices—and none of the doctors even knows for sure what they are."

"And every time you meet someone who's done it differently," I echoed her eagerly, "you're terrified that she or her doctor knows something your doctor doesn't."

I discovered in the months ahead that like almost all cancer patients, I tended to hear and remember cases that confirmed the validity of the forms of treatment I'd chosen. Later still, I learned to live more peacefully with ambiguity and uncertainty—as indeed everyone, healthy or sick, must do.

Sitting in the armchair, studying the newspaper clippings, I thought about how things have changed. Feminists and newspaper pundits tell you to take control of your treatment when you're ill. Cancer experts concur that patients who do this have the best prognosis. You should pull the doctor down from his godlike pedestal and quiz him, say these experts, get second opinions, read widely, make your own decisions. I'd always assumed that was good advice. Now it rang hollow. I had a week to decide about surgery. After that, there'd be a horde of other decisions. How could I possibly absorb enough information in that time, from my scraps of paper, my fevered phone conversations, to second-guess Dr. Day, who'd spent his life submerged in these issues? I appreciated his willingness to share his thoughts and doubts with me. But I was terrified by his youth, his vulnerability, his occasional awkwardness.

I longed for the all-knowing figure of television and movies. I longed for Dr. Kohn, the doctor I'd had as a child. On the way home from school, I'd peer into his window and, if the waiting room was empty, run in for a quick visit. He'd show me pictures in his medical books of germs and viruses and human organs, cheerfully check out any problem, from an infected pimple to a vague ache, give me one of the sweets he'd hung from the branches of a little metal tree on his table. I remembered how once a visitor to our house had fainted; we'd never seen anyone faint before and had fallen into utter confusion. But then my mother called Dr. Kohn. Five minutes later he was in our doorway, worn black bag in hand, looming dark against the brightness of the sun, warm and solid and infinitely reassuring. Oh, how I wanted him now.

In some ways the medical profession has rushed to meet patients' demand for more control. Was this analogous, I wondered (perhaps a little sourly), to the way in which many men, realizing that their wives' demands for meaningful work translated into dual incomes, had learned to embrace at least that one aspect of feminism? Surely the compliance of so many doctors stemmed more from their relative helplessness in the face of cancer, their inability to predict the results of their own interventions, than from any new-found respect for their patients.

In addition to the decision-making, there was the simple task of getting through the days. My sleep was broken, sporadic. Every morning I woke to the momentary hope that I'd been having a nightmare. Every morning I realized again that I did have cancer. And every morning I cried. Sometimes—when Bill and Anna were safely out of the house—I wailed and howled and cursed aloud. When the spasms were over, the cancer remained.

Intermittently, I thought about suicide. I believe most cancer patients do. Many healthy people, too, who have watched someone dying of cancer, have surely vowed, "I'll never go through this. I'll kill myself first."

I wasn't thinking about suicide in a sustained, reasonable way. The images came in flashes. I'd be driving down the street and would think about crossing the center line into the path of an oncoming truck. Only it seemed unfair to involve someone else. More responsible simply to drive off a cliff. But there was Anna. How could she possibly understand such an action?

At any rate, I wasn't very serious. I was waiting to see how things turned out. I figured there must be a trick to an effective suicide. You don't want to do it too soon and lose even a day of infinitely desirable life. And you don't want to wait until you're an object, the still center of a web of tubing, and couldn't take your own life if you wanted to.

Lynn had given me a relaxation tape, and one evening I turned it on and lay down on the living room carpet to listen. The voice was male, a little actorish, textured like the fur of a deep brown, well-hugged teddy bear. I learned later that it belonged to healer Emmett Miller. The voice gave instructions and praised me for following them with a warmly drawn-out "Gooood." At first I found it sappy, then seductive.

Miller led me through several imaginary scenarios: a trip downward in an ornate and luxurious elevator; a walk through peaceful woods; a confrontation with a mirror, during which I was to affirm my wholeness and perfection and put on whatever garment most pleased me. I chose something floating and white that let the air visit my body. A few nights before doing this exercise, I had dreamed that the lump had reappeared in my breast. Now, drifting off to sleep after listening to the tape, I saw my breast whole and round again, the scar completely effaced.

23

So sleep returned. And I learned something else that helped. I had thought that a diagnosis of cancer would change one ineradicably, that if it ever happened to me, I'd transform instantly into someone morose and homebound and fragile. What I discovered was that, even in the first two or three weeks of shock and terror, I remained essentially myself. It was much harder than usual to get out of bed in the morning. Taking a bath and seeing the biopsy scar was a grim and immediate reminder of my own mortality—so much closer now than it had ever seemed before. And getting ready for work in the morning was like starting a run after several weeks of inaction: the first steps were lead-heavy. But as the day wore on, I found I could become engrossed in a project for many minutes at a time, still laugh, still worry—in fragments at least—about international events. At home at night, I still played with our three dogs, rolling the bigfooted, comical Airedales over and over on the carpet, burying my face in their warm, hairy stomachs.

Sometimes when I picked up a kitchen knife to slice bread, a thought intruded, quick and sudden as a lizard's tongue: "Cut it off. Cut off your breast." It was a primitive urge, perhaps akin to that which causes a trapped animal to chew off the leg that threatens the survival of the entire body. And I think it was also a bid to prevent Dr. Day from cutting into me by doing it, however crudely, myself.

Surgery was set for Wednesday. On Tuesday, Bill and I returned to Dr. Susan Darcy's office. Officially, we wanted a second opinion about the surgery. But more than that, I hungered for the kindness, the steadying cool-headed honesty I remembered from our first visit.

Once again, we found ourselves seated in the small waiting room with the photographs of foxes and kittens on the walls, thumbing unseeingly through magazines. Only this time forty-five minutes went by before we were admitted to an examining room. Again we waited. Finally, Darcy appeared.

"I've studied the pathology report," she said, "and I agree with Dr. Day that a lumpectomy is sufficient. Only I think, if you were my patient, I'd go in and take out a little more tissue around the tumor. You had a clear margin, but it wasn't very big."

"And now," she added, "I really have to go. I'm due in surgery."

We struggled to detain her. "I ... I have some questions," I said.

She repeated, "I really have to go. However, there's a book by Lawrence LeShan called *You Can Fight for Your Life*. I recommend it to all my cancer patients."

She scribbled the title on a piece of paper.

I stepped forward as she started to walk out of the room. "Dr. Darcy, please, what do you think my prognosis is?"

She kept walking. "Impossible to tell," she said lightly over her shoulder. "It all depends on the lymph nodes." And she was gone.

We drove home in silence.

Still, there was no straw I wouldn't seize. The next day I picked up LeShan's book and put it aside to read later.

The day before the node dissection surgery, Bill and I visited the radiation center and spoke to the medical director, Dr. Norman Aarestad. A slender upright man with graying curly hair, a whimsical manner and the suggestion of a barely repressed chuckle behind his words, he leaned against the examining table in his white coat and talked to us, gesturing with the delicate hands of a pianist, listening carefully, never hurrying us, answering all our questions. After our experience with Dr. Darcy, we absorbed his patience and kindness with hungry gratitude. As we were walking out the door, he patted me on the shoulder. "Have fun tomorrow," he said.

It was almost puckishly unexpected. I had thought he'd say something serious, a grave "Good luck tomorrow" perhaps. For a second it redefined the coming ordeal. Charmed, I thought, well, yes, surgery will be an adventure.

Our next stop was at the office of the anesthesiologist. We walked across the street and entered the bowels of the Boulder Medical Center, where a nurse called Carol Marcoux spoke to me for a few minutes, telling me she'd be there to help me the next day, that I'd be able to leave by afternoon. Then Dr. Elizabeth Lou Lombard appeared in the doorway. I followed her into her office.

Lombard, who was black, had the warm, humorous, matter-of-fact kindness I associate with Jewish mothers. She told me about the combination of drugs she'd be using to put me to sleep. She said that when I was under she would slide a tube into my throat to breathe for me. I found that detail terrifying.

Some months earlier, my newspaper had printed an article on anesthesia. It said that, no matter how deeply asleep they were, many anesthetized patients could hear what was going on in the operating room, even if they never remembered it. The article described a woman who had woken up deeply depressed because the doctors had been joking about how fat she was, and other patients who on some level remembered derisive comments on their chances for survival and died soon after surgery in despair. Something like this had reportedly happened to Andy Warhol when he was brought to the hospital unconscious, after being shot by Valerie Solanas. After that experience, friends said he'd vowed never to enter a hospital again, for fear he'd die there. And indeed, he did die on his next hospital visit, following a heart attack.

I asked Dr. Lombard about all this.

"I wouldn't allow that kind of talk in my operating room," she said firmly.

"Actually," she went on, "Dr. Day has some kind of relaxation tape he uses. I don't usually believe in any of that stuff. My background's strictly empirical, strictly chemical. Still, he put those headphones on a patient last week, and it must have done something. All her vital signs stayed steady as a rock through the whole surgery."

Finally, I asked if I could take a Valium in the morning, just a little something to help me get from my house to the medical center.

"Girl," she said, "don't mess with Valium. I've got much better stuff for you here."

When I got home, I found a flower arrangement from a friend. The card said: "The flowers, too, are blessed." I was profoundly sentimental during this period. Kindness made me weep. I thought of every card and flower and good wish as a breath, a feather's weight for life on the great scale where it is weighed against death. I picked a peach-colored rosebud to take with me to the medical center.

Later, Bill stopped me as I was walking into the bedroom. "I know this is terrible timing," he said. "But I have to do it. I need you to sign your will. I've been asking you to do it for months."

I couldn't answer.

"Oh, come on, don't give me that stricken, you-think-I'm-going-to-die look." All of a sudden, he was yelling. "It's something I've been telling you and telling you has got to be done."

I lay down on the bed and pulled the covers over my head. I didn't seem able either to fight him or to appeal for mercy. Suddenly, the covers were ripped back and he was standing over me, red-faced, shouting, "Get up. Get up, goddammit. You're not just going to lie there and die."

Bill and I had been married for fifteen years. We understood each other's every gesture, expression and tone. So even as I told myself that I had every right to be furious with him, I knew that he was as afraid about the surgery as I was and that his outburst was prompted by pain. I also understood that it was almost unendurable for someone as strong and active as Bill to be faced with a problem that he couldn't fix, couldn't even attack directly. He left the room, came back a few minutes later to apologize. His lips against my hair, he said, "I'm just so afraid of losing you."

Later we decided to go out for dinner. We went to a restaurant run by local followers of a spiritual leader known as Rudrananda. I had always found this place soothing, with its soft guitar music, muted, tasteful furnishings, Indian tapestries and Thai figurines: smiling, vengeful or meditative. Now I was so jittery that I simply couldn't sit at the table. I left, pacing the parking lot while Bill had our just-ordered dinners packed up to go.

That night, Bill made love to me, very slowly and gently. Under his hands, my body, from which I had felt numbly disassociated all week, began to breathe again. When he kissed the scar on my right breast, it was as if a healing rain were falling on a parched field. I think we both cried. But afterward—miraculously—I slept deeply and sweetly.

The next morning we drove Anna to school. There was a game the kids were playing around that time: when they saw a Volkswagen Beetle, they'd punch whoever was nearest on the arm and yell "Slug bug yellow" or "Slug bug blue." Anna and I played loudly all the way from our house to her school. After we'd dropped her off, Bill and I lapsed into silence.

At the medical center, I changed into a gown and some strange white surgical stockings. Then I lay down on a gurney and waited. Carol was very kind. She told me that they'd just finished operating on a two year old, and I shouldn't get upset if I heard crying. How unfair for such a little one to need surgery, I thought. I was afraid to ask what was wrong with the two year old; I was afraid to hear a child's crying. It seemed that a cry was all it would take to send me flying into a million tiny fragments.

Dr. Day came in. I noticed he was wearing wooden meditation beads. Earlier we'd seen a photograph of Muktananda in his office. He examined my chest, tapped the pads of his fingers on my back. "I'm afraid, Dr. Day," I said against his chest. "Yes," he said very softly, "I know. I know."

He finished his examination and seized the newspaper: "Hey, here's your horoscope. It says that you're going to have an adventure today."

I remembered my reaction to Dr. Aarestad's words. "Give me the newspaper," I said. "I don't believe it."

It was true.

But then Day and Carol left, and I was lying on the gurney, undistracted, staring at a round clock on the wall. Bill sat by me, reading. My teeth started to chatter. I could actually hear them clicking. Why didn't they give me the wonderful drug that had preceded the biopsy? Dr. Day returned with a small tape recorder and earphones. When he put them on me, I heard a rather prissy masculine voice telling me to relax, to be joyous, that the people around me had come to help. Oddly enough, it was reassuring.

Finally, they wheeled me into the operating room. The relaxation tape was still going—they played it continuously through the surgery, as it turned out. I saw Dr. Lombard hovering above me, smiling her comfortable smile—and then sweet oblivion.

When I drifted to consciousness, there was Bill's face, red-bearded, vital, welcoming. Carol was busy adjusting the intravenous drip. I was alive, and nothing seemed to hurt. I moved in and out of awareness for what seemed like a couple of hours.

Dr. Day had agreed with Darcy's recommendation. He had excised more tissue from the lumpectomy site, as well as taking out the lymph nodes. Now Dr. Lombard and Carol were adjusting the dressing over my breast. I had the hazy impression that Carol hadn't left my side since the surgery, hadn't allowed me to feel a second's discomfort.

"Will you look at that," said Dr. Lombard admiringly. "Will you look at the man's stitching?"

So Dr. Day was an artist of sorts. How sad, I thought, that the recipients of his handiwork should appreciate it so little. At first, anyway.

They gave Bill instructions for taking care of me. A tube had been attached under my arm, to drain the liquid usually absorbed by the lymph nodes. It culminated in a bulb in which fluid collected. Bill was to measure this three times a day. When the draining ceased, the tube could be removed.

Finally, they said I could go home and helped me into a wheelchair. "You did beautifully," said the orderly, trundling the chair down the corridor. "Breathing, heartbeat, everything—you never faltered for a moment." Dr. Lombard came running up behind us. She hugged me. "I hope you're going to be fine," she said. "I hope everything's great. You're just too damn healthy to be sick."

3
MORTALITY AND JOY

At home that afternoon, I was euphoric. Comfortably ensconced in a big armchair, my arm safely tucked against my side, not quite alert enough to read or focus on the television, I smiled vaguely at the dear familiar clutter all around me—the piles of books and newspapers, the music books scattered on the lid of the piano, the cards and flowers that littered the living room. At around four, Kathryn Bernheimer, the film reviewer from the newspaper, came by carrying a large cardboard box.

"Everyone in the department got together and talked about what to get you," she said. "We decided you probably had enough flowers. But we figured you wouldn't be up to cooking. So here's your dinner for the next few days."

The box was full of gourmet items from Alfalfa's, the local natural foods supermarket: pasta with shrimp, cheese, apple-raspberry juice, crisp, buttery almond cookies from Belgium.

There was a card, too, signed by everyone in the department. "Where's the index?" Cynthia Wahl, our beautiful and unconventionally stylish art director, had written teasingly—referring to the piddling little job on the Sunday magazine that I hated the most. "No problem. I'll make something up." "Be strong," wrote Kathryn, "take comfort in the fact that you are loved." Get well, come back soon, said everyone else. "Whoopie—ti-yi-yo. Git back (and git well) little filly," was John Lehndorff, the food editor's contribution, while David Menconi, the rock critic, wrote, "Please, baby, please, please, please, please, etc. etc. GET WELL SOON." The card made me cry.

The day slipped pleasantly away. At night I was grateful to discover that, despite the fact that I had to keep my right arm clamped firmly to my side, it wasn't difficult to find a comfortable position in our bed. The only problem was that I had to face away from Bill, and we generally sleep spoon fashion, his back curved companionably against my front.

On the second day, I tried reading Toni Morrison's *Beloved*. I got about twenty pages into it, and then the anguish in the book became unendurable. I set *Beloved* aside, promising myself I'd return to it when I felt stronger. Then I rummaged around for something more peaceful. And there on my shelf, I saw E. F. Benson's *Mapp and Lucia*.

As if I were slipping into a warm bath, I entered this quiet, torpid little world, this English seaside town perennially preoccupied with only one question: who will emerge as the reigning queen of local society: game, schoolgirlish Elizabeth Mapp or the indefatigable Emmeline Lucas, also known as Lucia. I lost myself happily in talk of local fetes and garden produce and little evenings of Mozart, all described in Benson's inimitable, gossipy style.

But anxiety was beginning to tinge the agreeable dopiness and emotional abdication of this swimmy time. On Friday I would discover the state of my lymph nodes. I knew that if they were unaffected by the cancer, I had perhaps a 90 percent chance of living out a normal life span. If they were cancerous, my chances plummeted.

Through Friday morning I kept hoping that Candis, Dr. Day's nurse, would call. She'd been so empathetic, I was sure that if the news were good, she wouldn't force me to wait until afternoon to hear it. But the phone was silent. At two, I found myself again in Dr. Day's small waiting room, Bill beside me, trying to concentrate on the shiny pages of a *Time* magazine. Finally, I was ushered into the examining room and given a robe. Dr. Day came in.

"We took out thirty-two lymph nodes," he told me carefully. He paused a fraction of a second, not looking at me. "And one of them was involved."

How he must hate giving out such news. I found I was having difficulty breathing, and he became visibly agitated. This must be how it feels to faint, I was thinking in some wonder, as my chest constricted so that the breath seemed unable to reach my lungs.

I remembered the visitor who had fainted at our house, and a girl in grammar school who had once collapsed in class. In general, fainting had always seemed the province of less hardy souls than myself.

Day pressed me back onto the examining table, and Bill took my hand. Candis ran from the room, came back in with a small can of grapefruit juice and handed it to me. My senses cleared sufficiently for me to hear Dr. Day saying, "One node may mean that some cells have escaped and there's a tumor forming somewhere else in your body. Or it may mean that your immune system has dealt with the cancer and you're clear."

I asked about my chances for survival. He responded that statistics are meaningless. That frightened me more. He sat down beside me, took my hand, seemed to be fumbling for words of comfort. "Look, we are all creatures of light," he said finally. "All of us are made of light."

In my mind, I saw again the boot touching down on the mountain ledge. But now the ledge was slippery with mud. The boot shifted and began to slide.

"You'll need to go and see the oncologist, Dr. Fleagle," Day told me when I was dressed and sitting in his office again.

"What'll he do?"

"Well, I talked to him about your case, and I know he's going to offer you adjuvant therapy."

Chemotherapy. Cecile had been on chemotherapy. She'd talked of nausea and weariness. The one thing she'd been able to eat during those weeks, she told me on our last visit, was some homemade plum jam I'd given her. As she described it, the medication made her feel as if she were filled with wet clay, and the jam's edge of sourness had cut through the clayey taste.

Chemotherapy hadn't helped her a whit. And years earlier, watching its effects on my dying mother, I had learned to think of it as a form of torture devised to torment cancer patients during their precious last months on earth.

The next Monday, wearing a gown, holding a little green-patterned paper cup of water, I waited for John Fleagle. I had fallen into the world of the sick, and it seemed my days were now to be eked out in waiting rooms, the tenor of my thinking and dreaming defined by the words of doctors.

Bill sat with me. He had come for every doctor's visit, every procedure so far. His mere presence tended to ease my mind. But in addition, he was sometimes better able to assimilate what the doctors were saying than I was, so that later I could check what I'd understood against what he had heard. He charted a steady helping course, never pressuring me to accept one treatment over another, always available to discuss, question or confirm my choices.

We'd heard mixed reports about Dr. Fleagle. I'd been told he was the best oncologist in town, a caring man who'd cured many cancer patients, kept others alive for longer than expected. I knew that he'd taken good care of Cecile when she was dying and allowed her to dictate the amount of morphine she required. By contrast, my mother's doctor had avoided her deathbed and had been reluctant to prescribe sufficient painkiller. But another friend, the son of a cancer patient, had told us he disliked Fleagle intensely, finding him cold and uncaring.

Where John Day was tall and athletic, Fleagle was shorter, softer in contour, with thinning sandy-brown hair and a crinkling, good-humored face. And where Day frequently seemed to grope for the words he wanted and appeared to withhold information he thought might trouble his patient, Fleagle talked long, softly, freely and steadily.

He came right to the point. When the lymph nodes were involved, he said, the patient's chances of survival dropped from 90 to 50 percent. It was true there were other positive indicators in my case: the tumor had been well differentiated and the cells had tested estrogen and progesterone receptive. These factors augured well. However, neither of them was as telling as the existence of that cancerous lymph node.

"But only one out of thirty-two ... ," I protested.

"Statistically," said Fleagle, "there's no difference between one and three. If four or more are involved, prognosis worsens again."

He was therefore recommending a course of chemotherapy, a regimen that he said had been shown to raise survival rates to around 70 percent, according to studies by the Italian breast cancer expert, Dr. Gianni Bonadonna. Most chemotherapies these days consist of a combination of drugs, rather than simply one agent, he told me. Mine was to be no exception. The drugs involved were Cytoxan, Methotrexate and 5-Fluorouracil; the protocol was known as CMF.

What about Adriamycin, the drug that had been given to my mother and to Cecile?

"Well," Fleagle responded, "we do know that Adriamycin is the strongest anticancer drug known. But it has its drawbacks. The side effects are much harder on the body; the drug can damage the heart, and a patient can only tolerate a certain amount of Adriamycin in a lifetime: once you've used up your allocation, so to speak, you can't use Adriamycin again."

However, some doctors do believe that it's most effective to throw the hardest punch early in treatment, and that theory is currently being tested, he explained. So if I would like to go on an experimental protocol involving Adriamycin, he could arrange it for me. The Adriamycin would be administered three times, over a three-month period. My reaction to it would doubtless be more violent than to the CMF, but the experience would also be over sooner. If I chose the CMF, I would receive treatment over a six-month period, during which I'd alternate, spending two weeks on the drugs, then two weeks off them.

Which did he recommend?

He was comfortable with either, but the numbers hadn't yet been compiled for the Adriamycin. The drug may offer an incremental increase in survival rates. But it may not. The figures on the CMF were in, and they seemed to be very good.

Another dilemma. Leanne, the acquaintance of my stepfather who had called the night after my first visit with Day, believed that it was the willingness of the M.D. Anderson Cancer Research Center to prescribe Adriamycin that had saved her life. But I had seen the drug's action on my mother, and it terrified me. Nor had it seemed to help her in the slightest.

"Your mother shouldn't have had Adriamycin," Dr. Fleagle

said when I mentioned it to him. "I can't imagine why they prescribed it. It's of no use for colon cancer at all."

"Fine," I thought, remembering my mother's bald head and shrunken face, the flood of brown vomit on the sheets of her hospital bed. "So they were experimenting. Now who's going to tell her they're sorry they were wrong?"

Fleagle's nurse, Patti Kealiher, had joined us. She was a tall young woman with an athletic, western look about her.

"The CMF isn't too bad," she told me, and the brisk kindness of her voice inspired instant trust. "Most of our patients feel a little sick; some say it's sort of like morning sickness, if you've ever been pregnant."

I'd floated through my pregnancy in an ecstatic mist. This sickness, however, would not be a proud badge of fertility, but a sign of something gone terribly wrong, of a failing and aging body.

"About sixty percent of our patients lose their hair," Patti went on. "Forty percent don't. You might be lucky."

I told Dr. Fleagle I'd want a second opinion, but we'd probably go with the CMF. "Fine," he responded. "We'll set a date in two weeks, to give you time to recover from the surgery."

Meanwhile, what about the radiation that is supposed to accompany a lumpectomy?

"Because of the affected lymph node," he said, "we'd like to do the chemotherapy first. After that, you'll go back to Dr. Aarestad for eight weeks of radiation."

Everything I read told me that breast cancer rates were surging. I asked Dr. Fleagle if he knew why. "Nobody really has an explanation," he responded.

"Could it be the birth control pill?" I had taken the pill for seven years in my twenties.

"No correlation has been found."

We went home to assimilate what we'd heard. I was beginning to understand some things about surgery. I had awoken from the operation filled with joy and gratitude for being alive. This response was not unusual. I learned later that patients were often

35

cheerful and talkative after even major surgeries. It seemed to take a few days for the body to realize fully the depth of the insult it had sustained. Then depression set in. Body and mind shrank from touch.

The drain under my arm troubled me. While it didn't hurt, it chafed constantly, and that, combined with my inability to raise my right arm, made simple tasks like taking a bath or washing my hair difficult. I took to wearing Bill's old shirts: they were soft and roomy enough to hide the tubing. I also believed they were somehow impregnated with his abundant vitality.

As post-surgical therapy, Bill insisted that I should go for walks with him and even try to swing my right arm a little as we walked. Our favorite path was by a stream. The trees we passed seemed so solid and strong that I wanted to press my body against them. The sunlight shimmered on the water.

I was continuing to see Dr. Wood every week, and I thought of a metaphor he had used once, of the mind as a powerful horse that we had to—not exactly control—but somehow work with. He'd pointed out to me that nothing the doctors had done to me after my diagnosis had been as painful as the thoughts and images I myself had conjured up. Almost all the pain was caused by my mind, by how I reacted to what was happening. The key, then, lay in healing the mind.

I'd liked the horse metaphor. It made me think of warm flanks and gentle breathing. But as I walked with Bill by the creek, the horse became a huge stallion, its sides wet, its nostrils wide with terror and rage. I felt that it would bolt at any moment, throw me to the ground, crush me under blindly thrashing hooves.

Once home, I called Dr. Wood. He again told me to create a schedule and stick to it, to do whatever work I had to do meticulously and with dedication.

"Routine," he said patiently, "is the tether for your stallion."

My sessions with Dr. Wood were becoming a lifeline. Because he was a foreigner like me (I'd grown up in England); because he understood, as my Central European parents had taught me, how a normal, middle-class life can suddenly collapse into sheer horror; most of all, because his slight accent, wry smile, slender build and dark hair all reminded me irresistibly of my father, I felt a powerful bond with him.

He was teaching me something that seemed oddly paradoxical: you can deal with despair and the fear of death by sharpening your senses, allowing yourself to be fully absorbed in the sights, sounds, smells and feel of each precious and specific moment of living. In other words, in the face of death, you are strengthened by immersing yourself in those very things—the evidence of your faculties, the presence of loved ones, natural beauties—that death will take away from you.

I once interviewed a Salvadoran refugee for my newspaper. He had been through a great deal, from fighting and almost starving in the mountains to torture at the hands of the Honduran government. He recounted all this with great vivacity and odd, gallant flashes of humor. "I was a dragon," he said, describing how he'd thrown up after electric shock torture. "I was a dragon shooting fire from my mouth."

After three days of torture, they came for him at four in the morning. He believed he was going to be shot. And I kept remembering his next words: "You have no idea," he'd said, with a kind of aching intensity, "how beautiful a street can look when you know you're about to die."

Dr. Wood is from Chile. He has seen people die, both as a doctor and during the 1973 coup in his country. He never tried to dissuade me from talking about death, and he never substituted platitudes about holding to positive thoughts for honest discussion. This was as refreshing as a long drink of water on a hot day.

He told me that when a patient is near death, the mind disassociates from the body. If the dying process is grievous or panicky, it is because of the images the patient has conjured up.

We discussed an Aldous Huxley novel I'd read once, in which one of the protagonists finds himself after death, floating in the void. He's desperate to become one with the eternal, the great light. But he can't give up the world: he's holding on to a fragment of a Mozart concerto, playing it over and over in his mind. And

37

those few bars of music tie him to the material, prevent his apotheosis. (I remember at the time thinking this extraordinarily ironic. It seemed if anything could facilitate an entrance to heaven, it would be Mozart. But I supposed that was Huxley's point.)

If Huxley's vision is true, there's not much hope for me, I told Antonio Wood. I have been so passionately in love with the things of this earth: daffodils, apple trees, coffee, sex, the smell of my daughter's skin and hair. It was unthinkable to lose them.

And when the mind unravels, I wondered, what happens to all the silly jokes we know, the places and faces we've memorized, the snatches of song, the precious little store of knowledge, even wisdom we've so painstakingly accumulated?

After death, would I be able to stay by Anna, to watch over her as she entered the perilous years of puberty? In my mind I promised that I would always be with her, but then I wondered if that was true. Or rather, since it simply had to be, in what sense it was true.

Just in case no vestige of individual consciousness does survive death, I thought, what could I leave to protect and comfort her? A journal, a videotape, a joke on my tombstone?

My mind beat against the finality of death like a trapped bird hurling itself against a window.

On Friday evening—a week and a half after my surgery—I went to see Anna in *Coppelia*. She was one of four children who danced onto and across the stage at intervals in the action. Normally, seeing Anna dance is one of my purest and most intense pleasures. This time I couldn't concentrate. The auditorium was astonishingly cold for a pleasant May evening, my arm ached, I wanted desperately to go home. After the performance, there were perfunctory hugs and congratulations, and Anna left with friends for a cast party. I was noticing that my inability to deal with her directly seemed to be matched by her desire not to have to face me. It was as if we were rehearsing for a possible forced separation.

On Saturday morning I woke up in a panic to find my side drenched with liquid. "My God," I thought, "I'm spilling." The lymph fluid was slipping down the sides of the drain instead of through it. Bill took me to the emergency room at the medical center. There I was shown into yet another examining room. Suddenly I was crying. These weren't the passionate tears I had shed a week or two ago. This was the kind of hopeless grizzling you hear from a child who's too dejected and beaten down even to wipe the snot from her nose. It was all too much. I had cancer. I was weak. I was afraid they were going to hurt me.

"I'm sorry to be such a crybaby," I told the young intern who came in, with a nurse, to check on me.

"That's all right," he said. "A diagnosis of cancer is just about the worst thing that can happen to anyone." Neither Day nor Fleagle would ever have said anything like that (they are probably all too well aware that there are worse things), and I was a little taken aback. Comforted, too, in an odd way, that a doctor had acknowledged my pain as legitimate.

The doctor and the nurse entered into a hurried consultation. They called Dr. Day, who apparently gave them instructions. I was afraid they would remove the tube and replace it, and that would hurt. But they only pulled a long string of clotted blood from it. "Aha," said the doctor. "Here's the problem." He left the room, the nurse replaced the irritating wet dressings under my arm with clean, dry bandages and I began to feel better.

"I know just what you're going through," she said kindly. She hesitated a moment, then said in a lower voice, "I have a lump in my breast. They're not sure what it is, but they want to watch it for a while. In four months they'll examine me again."

I could sense her fear, and I knew my part in this dialogue by heart. "It's probably nothing at all," I said. I was, of course, reiterating what she already knew. "Nine times out of ten those lumps aren't cancer." She touched my shoulder, and we smiled at each other. It wasn't clear who was comforting whom.

One thing I could still do, even though I couldn't raise my arm, was play the piano. I was no virtuoso. It was just that when Anna had started piano lessons a couple of years earlier, I had begun remembering my childhood teacher and growing increasingly envious. Finally, I'd decided to take lessons, too.

39

The drain dangling by my side, I fumbled through Beethoven's "Moonlight Sonata." I noted that even though I was playing badly, the music seemed to come through, crowding between the awkwardly pressed keys as though it had an existence independent of my fingers. No matter how many notes I blurred, it was still indisputably Beethoven, still indisputably the "Moonlight."

So I'd found a sense in which death wasn't final. These musical shapes had been created by a genius. And even though the brain that had formed them had long since rotted away, they survived, to unfurl themselves in my living room.

I was planning to return to work the next Monday and had hoped to have the drain out by then. However, Saturday's emergency had shown that quantities of fluid were still draining. I knew that a possible consequence of lymph node removal was a painful, swelling condition called lymphedema, and I kept nervously closing the fingers of my left hand around the flesh of my upper arm, trying to determine whether it was becoming bulbous, imagining liquid trapped there.

I had a practical problem. The comfortable men's shirts I'd been wearing were hardly suitable for work. I mentioned this to Bill on Sunday night. "Hold on," he said, "I think I may have a solution." He left the room. A few minutes later he was back, holding a silky garment: golden-brown crescents floated on a background of tiny green squares.

"It's a Japanese robe," he said. "I got it when I was eleven, when Dad was stationed in Japan. Try it on."

It was perfect, capacious. It fell to my hips, completely covering up the tubing and bulb. In the morning I put it on over a pair of pants, scrounged up a sash to keep it closed, and set off for work, driving as best I could with a right arm that refused to raise itself past half-mast.

"So," said Kathryn, as I walked into the department, "you weren't sick at all. You were just out shopping for that beautiful top."

Being at work was a great relief. It gave some shape and semblance of normalcy to my days, even though I tended to be forgetful of details. The people in my department were warmly supportive and helpful in covering my deficiencies. One morning the art director, Cynthia Wahl, presented me with a little gold box containing an outrageous pair of earrings. They were made of some lightweight foil—each a swirl of pink covered with smudges of green, purple and blue. They were unlike anything I'd ever buy for myself. They were wonderful.

Later in the week, Bill and I decided to attempt another evening out, this time with our friends. Donovan, whose "Mellow Yellow" and "Jennifer Juniper" had been big hits in the sixties, was coming to Boulder to perform at the Chautauqua, a huge wooden concert hall. Lynn and Gunner were going, as well as two other couples, Steve and Louise Silvern and John and Douchka Dingler. All our children, one daughter apiece, were with us. As we settled in our seats, Douchka was telling me about an accident she'd had at work. She had spilled a cup of boiling coffee down her front, creating a huge, painful burn over her breastbone. She was laughing about it now, but for a few days it had been anything but a laughing matter. The two of us looked down the row. Louise was suffering from injuries she'd sustained in a car accident over a year earlier. Her cane rested by her seat. Lynn was still struggling to cope with the death of Cecile. We were, the four of us agreed ruefully, a pathetic group of women.

Slowly the drafty wooden auditorium filled with people, chatting, hugging acquaintances, bringing with them breaths of the sweet summer air. I thought about the way I'd always bragged to out-of-town friends about how beautiful Boulderites are: "You have to stay active to live in this town," I'd kid. "There's a city ordinance, and they throw out people who don't stay in shape." After my years of living in big cities, watching pallid people scurry through grimy streets, I loved walking on the Boulder Mall, watching the flat bellies and muscled thighs of young people in shorts and skimpy T-shirts. Even the old people here seemed vigorous, clear-eyed and slender, with the easy gait of long-distance walkers. But suddenly the robustness of the others in the auditorium, their tanned fleshiness, seemed like an assault. Holding myself in tight, cradling my hurt arm to my body, I felt a huge gulf separating me from these people. They seemed so strong and so very alive.

The warm-up performer for Donovan, a self-conscious young man singing folk songs, didn't help. During these early months after diagnosis, it seemed dangerous for me to get into any situation—a long car trip, a movie that wasn't utterly absorbing—where I had to sit and do nothing for an hour or two. On these occasions, I couldn't avoid my fears. As I had in the restaurant the night before surgery, I jittered silently, cursing the long minutes, yearning to go home.

Then Donovan was onstage, and the first bars of "Mellow Yellow" were filling the auditorium. I was amazed at his authority as a musician, the complexity and lyricism of his guitar playing. I'd liked him well enough in the sixties, but now he seemed infinitely better. Surrounded by the wistfully joyous sounds of "Jennifer Juniper," I leaned against Bill's shoulder, smiling and clapping. Douchka glowed with pleasure, the men in the group beamed. Sixties waifs that we all were, we had come home.

On Friday, I went to Dr. Day to get the tube removed. I had taken Valium again that morning. I assumed that the procedure couldn't hurt much, but I seemed oversensitized to even the possibility of pain. I remembered my mother telling me how she'd become afraid to go to the dentist after her surgeries. "It's ridiculous," she'd said, laughing, "I know having my teeth cleaned or getting a filling is so minor compared to what I've been through. You'd think it wouldn't matter at all. But it's just the opposite. I can't bear the thought of the dentist poking in my mouth. I just can't bear having anything done to me."

Dr. Day came in and told me I was looking well. He fidgeted a second, and suddenly the irritating tube that had been chafing the soft skin of my underarm for almost two weeks was out. It happened so fast and painlessly that I didn't realize it was gone for a moment. I thought that he had only cut off the bottom half.

"There you go," he said.

Again, a state of lightness and joy. Slowly, I was beginning to understand something important. I didn't know if I'd live six more months or forty more years, but then I hadn't known that before—and neither did anyone else. I felt as if I, with nine-tenths of the population, had been sleepwalking all this time: repeating meaningless routines, spooning food into our unblinking faces, watching television, completely unaware of the abyss yawning beneath our feet.

The newspapers are routinely full of unexpected deaths: two women set out in a perky yellow car and are crushed against the side of a mountain by a runaway truck; a father and daughter are swept away at sea during a summer vacation; a group of passengers, laughing and chatting, boards an airplane that harbors a bomb.

When—at last—you fully believe in your own mortality, you regain the sense of wonder, the ability to lose yourself completely in the moment, that you had as a child. As I left work at night, I'd marvel at the deepening green of the trees across the street from the parking lot. Each day the sky seemed more extraordinarily vivid, the tracery of branches against it more beautiful, the people I loved dearer.

I thought of some lines from one of Shakespeare's sonnets: "This thou perceivest, that makes thy love more strong / To love that well which thou must leave e'er long."

And I remembered a tiny old lady I'd seen once on the downtown mall. She was standing in the middle of the sidewalk, in a lacy white dress and a broad-brimmed hat, as prim and pretty as a little girl about to take communion. And she was gazing around wide-eyed, astonished, storing everything up.

As I watched her, I knew that she was dying. She must have been housebound for a while, I reasoned, and this morning her caretakers had helped her up and dressed her, and she'd asked to go out alone for one last foray into the world. So there she was. Motionless. Drinking in every movement of the wind, the people strolling by absorbed in their own concerns, the scent of the summer air, the grass and flowers, the whole infinitely precious world.

"Congratulations," said Dr. Wood, when I told him of these revelations at our next session. "I see you're finally awake."

4
CHEMOTHERAPY

I'd decided to go to Dr. Jennifer Caskey of the AMC Cancer Research Center in Lakewood, a twenty-minute drive from Boulder, for a second opinion on the chemotherapy. I'd heard of her through our film reviewer Kathryn, whose cousin worked at the center.

That morning, at Candis's direction, I went to Boulder Community Hospital to pick up the slides of my tumor. I was handed a large cardboard tube. As I turned from the desk I saw a corpse sliding by on a gurney. At least I thought it was a corpse. The man's mouth was open, he had the gray pallor of death on his skin, he brought with him the depthless hush that always seems to accompany the flight of the soul. An elderly woman and a middle-aged couple walked alongside the gurney, which was pushed by a young male orderly. No one wept. No one spoke. The members of the little group carried their freight of silence with them, disappearing like a cold breath, down the corridor and out of sight.

The wait for Dr. Caskey was long. I sipped the herb tea the research center had kindly provided and began to wonder why we'd come. Dr. Fleagle seemed completely trustworthy, the regime he'd recommended uncontroversial. I was also afraid that Caskey would prescribe a different protocol. Getting a second opinion seemed to be a good general principle, but what did you do with it once you had it? How did you decide which doctor was right? Finally, after filling in some forms, I again found myself swathed in a paper robe on an examining table. Jennifer Caskey, a small woman with soft brown hair, entered, asked a few questions in a gentle voice, began touching me. Some patients resent these endless examinations, but I always found them reassuring—even though I knew full well what the doctors were feeling for. I seemed to gentle at the touch of a good doctor the way our dogs do when the vet places his hands on them—wary, yet oddly at peace.

I'd also noticed, over the last few weeks, that every doctor had a specific and individual way of communicating with my body. John Day probed with straight hard fingers in some places, rolled the flesh gently back and forth in others; Dr. Fleagle's touch took in a greater area and was lighter—though there were one or two places where he, too, pressed hard. Jennifer Caskey seemed to bring the deepest concentration to the task. She moved her soft little fingers over my back and across my chest, silent, her head to one side. She seemed to be listening as well as feeling for messages from my body. She asked questions nobody else had asked. Why were my hands peeling? I didn't know; I thought it was nerves. Had I ever smoked? Yes, I responded, with a stab of guilt. For a long time. I had quit fifteen years earlier.

"Good for you," she said warmly.

When she touched the scar on my breast, I began to cry.

"I'm sorry," she said, stopping immediately. "Does it hurt?"

I shook my head. I couldn't explain.

"This is the worst thing that's ever happened to you, isn't it?" she said. "You've always been strong and healthy, and now this—it just doesn't make any sense."

I felt a tremendous surge of affection for her.

Afterward we talked. She congratulated me on having gone to a doctor when I'd first felt the lump. "You may have saved your life," she said. To my relief, she recommended the same chemotherapy Dr. Fleagle had, only suggesting that, in the last couple of months, it be administered in conjunction with the radiation so as to shorten the overall treatment time. (Fleagle and Aarestad considered this approach, but eventually decided it would be too debilitating.) Caskey also amended Fleagle's estimate that chemotherapy gave me a 70 percent chance of five-year survival.

"I think," she said, "since only one out of thirty-two lymph nodes was involved, and since you're relatively young and very healthy, it might be a little higher than that. Somewhere around eighty-five percent perhaps."

There was one more interesting fact. I associated chemotherapy with emaciation. But Dr. Caskey told me that many people on the regime I would be following gained weight. I felt simultaneously relieved and aggrieved.

"Wonderful," I said to Bill once we'd left Caskey's office. "I'm not only gonna be bald, I'm gonna be fat. I hope your sexual fantasies include sleeping with Telly Savalas."

Nevertheless, he was smiling as we settled into the car. "We had to wait a while," he said, "and the place seemed a little disorganized. But hey"—and he reached across for my hand—"Jennifer Caskey was great. And I like her statistics. This was one trip that was worth making."

I was happy, too. I had been impressed with the breadth of John Fleagle's knowledge. Now another, obviously first-rate physician had seconded his opinion. There seemed to be no need to go to Houston for treatment.

I tried to prepare for chemotherapy in every way possible. In Bernie Siegel's book, *Love, Medicine and Miracles*, he showed a drawing made by a patient who, he said, would clearly not profit much from her treatments. In the drawing, a tube enters the arm of a melancholy figure. But everything stops at the barrier of skin, nothing seems to enter the body. What was needed, apparently, was a positive visualization: the woman should have seen the chemicals as something like a stream of sunlight, flowing into her, penetrating every cell, bringing healing and wholeness.

Creating such images was going to take work. Since reading Rachel Carson's *Silent Spring* in the sixties, I had been appalled by the industrialized world's dependence on chemicals. I had sought out organic produce for my family, refused to eat foods containing dyes, flavorings or preservatives, argued Bill out of spraying insecticide to eliminate house ants. Hell, we even used organic toothpaste. Now I was proposing to flood my system with chemicals known to attack the bone marrow; impair the functioning of the immune system; kill all dividing cells, healthy along with cancerous; and quite possibly cause leukemia or other forms of cancer.

I read the pamphlets on chemotherapy nurse Patti Kealiher had given me on my last office visit. It seemed that Fluorouracil and Cytoxan (or cyclophosphamide) could cause blood in the urine; dizziness, confusion or agitation; fever; sores in the mouth and on the lips; black, tarry stools; yellow eyes and skin. Methotrexate could have some of the same side effects, as well as causing stomach pain and bloody vomit. Symptoms that could be caused by all three drugs and did not require medical treatment— that were, in other words, expected—included weakness, loss of appetite, loss of hair, nausea and vomiting. Earlier, Dr. Fleagle had said that, at my age, chemotherapy would probably put an end to my periods.

I had found a tape containing visualizations for chemotherapy in a local bookstore. Now I stretched out on the living room carpet to listen to it. The narrator suggested I imagine myself by a river: "Just being here, in this lovely setting, enables you to relax ... breathing in a gentle flow of harmony, balance and deep peace. ... The warm sunlight against your forehead helps you to feel at peace. ... The sunlight warms your body. ... Simply being here at this lovely river is very healing. ... As you sit in your chair, you are able to listen to the soft breeze whistling through the trees. ... It's so soothing, and very calming for you. ..." And on and on.

I endured about five minutes of this, but the editor in me was outraged by the repetition (some repetition, of course, is necessary on such tapes, to induce deep relaxation, but here there was no sense of progression or organization); the banality; the slipshod use of language (why would a soft breeze "whistle"?). The whole thing was, as we used to say in grammar school, soppy. I gave up and went back to the teddy-bearish Emmett Miller, whose soothing voice had helped me win back sleep.

I also selected some Mozart horn concerto music to play in the chemotherapy room. And then I called Sara Wolfe; Dr. Fleagle had given me her number when I asked to speak with someone else who'd been through chemotherapy.

Sara had had an aggressive and unclassifiable tumor, and doctors had given her no more than a 5 percent chance of survival. She had been treated with Adriamycin and now, four years later, was in good health. The treatments, however, had been devastating. She described nights of vomiting, days of nausea, the loss of all her hair. She also described the tenderness of a roommate who, no matter how quietly Sara crept to the bathroom at night, would appear beside her, hold her head as she vomited, wipe her face, bring her water. I'm not going to be on Adriamycin, I kept reminding myself as she spoke. This won't happen to me.

Eventually, I would come to know Sara better. For the moment—despite the dismaying descriptions—she served as reassurance that I would survive chemotherapy. And we shared our rage and confusion about what had happened to us.

"I've always been a health food fanatic," I told her. "Always jogged and exercised ... "

"Yes," she chimed in. "Me, too."

"And now I'm meeting all kinds of women like me who have breast cancer. It seems like it's a healthy woman's disease. And it's so unfair. You see all these people who smoke and drink and eat garbage and seem to survive into their nineties. You hear about old Mafia dons drifting peacefully into eternal sleep after a lifetime of swindling and having people killed ... "

"I know," said Sara. "Couldn't you just die?"

Simultaneously we realized what she'd said and burst out laughing.

Sara also told me how having cancer had changed her life, how she'd started doing the things she wanted to do: "It may sound silly, but I decided to take singing lessons. It's something I'd always thought about, but never done."

She was about to become the director of a Denver support organization called QuaLife. "You might want to attend some of our events," Sara said. "We have a three-day weekend coming up. It's great. There'll be workshops on nutrition and keeping a journal and visualization. ..."

While I struggled to get ready for chemotherapy, Anna suddenly asserted herself. It was a year before she could tell me how afraid she'd been the afternoon she came to my office and was told that I was seeing a doctor, there was something wrong with my mammogram. She understood what that meant. She had known Cecile, her almost-grandmother, well. Four weeks before the older woman's death, Anna had brought a tape of wistful piano music (I remembered its title as something like "Evening Bells") to her house, along with a gauzy ballet skirt and her soft pink slippers. She had danced for Cecile gravely on the living room carpet. Leaning back on the sofa, an uncharacteristically misty look about her eyes, Cecile had drunk her in.

My co-workers hadn't been sure how much to tell Anna. They had fumbled and prevaricated before John Lehndorff finally said: "Hey, she has a right to know. Anna, there was something wrong with your mom's mammogram. She's gone to see a doctor. But I'm sure she's going to be OK."

Then, in the weeks preceding surgery, I'd paid little attention to my daughter. I was afraid to face her. Her fear intensified mine. We couldn't look into each other's eyes without seeing the specter of losing each other. At least, I kept telling myself, she's ten; she's old enough to remember me if I die. I'll have had some influence on who she becomes. I myself had only the haziest memories of my father, who died when I was four.

Finally, she confronted me as I stacked the dishwasher in the kitchen. She needed information, she said. She needed to know everything that I was told during my endless round of doctors' offices. Not knowing was frightening—more frightening, even, than getting bad news. Humbled and impressed by her strength of will, her ability to articulate her needs, I promised that in the future I'd sit down and talk to her after every doctor's appointment and phone call.

Oh, and another thing, she said, I was thinking too much about all this. I was ruining the time we spent barbecuing with friends or listening to music, worrying. She could see me worrying. "Do what I do," she insisted. "Whenever the word *cancer*—

49

or anything else bad—comes up on this blackboard I have in my head, I just wipe it away. I get rid of it and write down something good."

I have since talked to other breast cancer patients about how they've dealt with their children. Twenty years ago, when the disease tended to strike only older women (and women generally had their babies earlier), it was rare for sufferers to have babies or small children in the house. Now—no one knows why—the disease is affecting younger and younger women. Some of these mothers have a great deal of difficulty communicating with their children; some even appear to reject them.

One morning, I saw a letter in the newspaper from a woman named Karen DuBose. She said she had a particularly deadly form of breast cancer—inflammatory carcinoma, as it turned out—and she called for the closing of the Rocky Flats weapons plant, which she believed might be the cause. She mentioned her two children.

I called to ask for an interview; Karen was friendly and open. But during the course of that phone conversation, I made an unforgivable gaffe. In the preceding weeks, I had found an immediate intimacy with other breast cancer victims and a tremendous honesty of expression. So when she told me that her oldest child was four at the time she was diagnosed and the youngest weeks old and still nursing, I said instantly and without thinking that that was terrible, that my father had died when I was four and I barely remembered him.

I lay awake that night cursing myself for the possibility that I had added, thoughtlessly, to the burden of someone who had an incurable cancer. It wasn't even true that I didn't remember my father, I berated myself. To be sure, I didn't remember much that was specific about him. But I had a clear sense of his courtesy and humor, of his loving presence.

When I arrived at her house the next day, however, Karen welcomed me and talked freely about the impact of her illness on her family. "I let things fall apart," she told me. "I didn't try to take care of the baby anymore. I didn't try to do the grocery shopping. And my four year old—I was sort of convinced that I actually might die then. I was that sick. And he would overhear conversations, and he got kind of withdrawn. ... My sister-in-law's been taking care of him a lot. ... So my one contact with him was at night. I'd put him to bed and I would read him a story, and we would talk about dying, what it meant to die. He would ask me, 'Are you going to die?' And I would never say, 'Yes.' I mean, I would say, 'Well, everybody does at some point,' and try to keep things in the present moment. But I think I may have scared him a little more than I needed to. I mean, I was so frightened myself."

As for the new baby, "I couldn't relate to her at all. My attention span was ... I couldn't even hold her. I was afraid I would drop her. I remember ... I tried to make a peanut butter and jelly sandwich for Michael, and it took me two hours. That's how disoriented I was.

"I didn't want her to get attached to me. And then my mother-in-law says, 'Look, look, she really loves you.' I'm like, 'No. Get her away from me. One more thing to let go of. Get her away.' Now," her voice softened, "she's my baby."

I prepared for the chemotherapy as Dr. Fleagle had suggested, taking Compazine, an antinausea pill, the night before my first session, as well as Xanax, a medication designed to quell anxiety in the morning. At quarter to three on a Wednesday afternoon, Bill picked me up at work and drove me to Fleagle's office.

I told Dr. Fleagle the pamphlets had frightened me, and he looked concerned. "None of those extreme things are likely to happen," he said. "They won't happen to you. But I'm ethically obliged to warn patients that they're a possibility. Can you think of a better way to do it?" I couldn't.

I soon came to know the routine of these visits by heart; it was, so to speak, engraved on my skin. Dr. Fleagle made a little calendar for me on a specially prepared sheet of paper marked off in white and pale purple squares. Two Wednesdays in a row I'd come in for injections of Methotrexate and Fluorouracil. Every day in between I'd take the Cytoxan by mouth: sometimes two pills, sometimes three, until the fourteen days were up. I'd get two weeks' respite and repeat the cycle.

Patti Kealiher was out of the office that first day, and a pleasant, plump young woman was slated to tend to me. She asked me to weigh myself, and then drew blood from the crook of my arm, making me wait while she tested it. This, I was to learn, was a regular part of the procedure. I could not receive chemotherapy unless my white blood count was above a certain level. Whenever the count slipped too far, treatment was postponed for a week. For this first treatment, however, my count was healthy, and I was taken into the chemotherapy room. This was a small, comfortable place, with magazines in racks, plants in the sunny window. Four huge armchairs were crowded into the room, and a smaller chair sat in attendance on each. Some kinds of chemotherapy take a long time to administer, I discovered, and patients sometimes sat in these chairs for four to six hours. The atmosphere was always quite placid. People read or chatted, idly flipped the pages of magazines, ignored the paraphernalia linking their throats or wrists to overhead bottles of caustic chemicals.

On this first visit, I was tense and afraid. The nurse turned on the Mozart for me, slipped the needle into a vein on the back of my left hand (with remarkable smoothness, I thought) and taped it down. She explained that they'd prefer never to inject anything into my right arm, because the node dissection had made it very vulnerable to infection. Then she proceeded to attach small tubes of different colored liquids, one by one, to the tubing going into my vein. First she injected Benedryl, which I came to call happy juice. It made me cheerful, dry-mouthed and talkative. Then came clear saline to clear the vein, Methotrexate, saline again, Fluorouracil and finally more saline. The saline burned a little going in.

While the nurse was working, a young woman came into the room for a shot. She winced and squeezed her eyes shut when she was pricked. I pounced on her like a clumsy, friendly puppy, making Benedryl-flavored conversation, and she confessed that she had a terror of needles. She also told me that she had a rare blood condition that could be controlled by the drug she had just taken. She seemed anxious to make it clear that she did not have any kind of cancer, and I sensed she wanted to distance herself from this room and its usual inhabitants. Who could blame her? After a few minutes she left, to be replaced by a young man who looked about thirty. I wondered at the relative youth of so many of Dr. Fleagle's patients.

The nurse's work with me took around ten minutes. She left, and Bill went to the desk to pay for the treatment. High on happy juice and indescribably relieved because the procedure was over, I babbled cheerfully to the dark-haired young man. He was very friendly, but I retained no memory of what he said. Then I followed Bill out to the desk area, where I hugged the nurse, who seemed a little surprised, and told her that she'd done a wonderful job. Once home, I roamed the house restlessly for half an hour or so, then collapsed on the bed and slept. I woke several hours later to a sick taste in the back of my throat. It was to be my companion, at varying levels of intensity, for the next six months.

My first reaction to the chemotherapy was that it wasn't nearly as bad as I'd expected. I didn't vomit. Despite the continual queasiness, I could function over the two-week period that I was on it: drive, work, make love, even eat. Many months later, after it was all over, the emotional effect seemed to hit me. I decided then that being on the CMF protocol is rather like being in the punishment machine Franz Kafka describes in his short story "The Penal Colony." The machine begins by tracing a description of the crime on the perpetrator's body. This is painless. Then the machine repeats the action. And repeats it. Over and over, imprinting the words ever deeper into the flesh, muscle, tissue and bone of the prisoner until he dies.

With the kind of chemotherapy I was on, the nausea was manageable. But it was all pervasive. You couldn't get relief by throwing up, because the irritant wasn't in your stomach or your bowels: it permeated your entire system. The pamphlets had described the taste the chemicals leave in your mouth as metallic, but that wasn't it, really. It was quite indescribable—a warm, sick, alien taste that I continually tried to wash down with water and orange juice but that flavored everything I ate and tainted the nature of my days. I became more and more aware over the months of how assiduously my body was working to expel the poison—only to be assaulted by it over and over again. The weariness this caused was mitigated by a kind of jagged speediness provided by the Cytoxan.

It wasn't that the effect of the drugs increased as the months went by. It was that my body seemed to recognize the enemy more quickly and to respond to it more strongly with each application. My veins closed up and scarred. Little bumps appeared on the back of my wrist. Visit by visit, it became increasingly difficult for Patti to slip the needle in.

"There's a constant seething inside you," I told Dr. Fleagle, trying to describe chemotherapy for a young resident he was escorting through his offices. "When I'm on it, I feel as if there's a witch's cauldron in my belly."

The evening after my first treatment, however, I awoke to the smell of dinner cooking. Bill was making baked chicken, mashed potatoes and spinach. Everything smelled wonderful, and I was filled with joy at my hunger, my ability to eat. Later I learned that the nausea came and went in unpredictable patterns. Sometimes I had to go into our bedroom and close the door while Bill cooked; the smell of cooking nauseated me, though I could usually eat once the food was ready. ("So handy for you," Bill used to mock. "Means you never have to get your ass in here and help out.")

The nausea didn't come at any particular time of day or any specific point in the drug cycle. It wasn't worse in the fourth month than in the first, though I seemed to react to it more strongly as time went by, and it did seem particularly acute on the days when I took three Cytoxan tablets instead of two. On some days, I ate large amounts. On others I picked listlessly at a chicken salad, afraid my inability to choke any of it down signaled the beginning of drug-induced anorexia. There were certain smells that triggered the sickness; we had to change our brand of dishwashing liquid, for instance, because every time I tried to wash dishes, I was reminded of Dr. Fleagle's office. Eventually, the saliva would gather in my mouth, and I'd find myself swallowing frantically if I merely heard Patti Kealiher's voice on the phone—an ungrateful response, I often thought, to her dedicated and empathetic nursing. In one of my books, there was an anecdote about a man who'd spotted his oncologist in a department store and had thrown up on the spot. Reading this before I'd had chemotherapy, I found it frightening. Afterward, I thought it was funny. How in the world did they explain the mess to the store manager?

Even typing these words, I can feel the familiar taste, the gorge rising in my throat.

I settled into the regime, and the tilt toward chaos that my life had taken began to even out. The chemotherapy weeks were quite endurable, the two weeks off invariably ecstatic. For six months I alternated between sickness and euphoria, the way you walk through sunlight and shadow on a pathway flanked by pillars.

Anna seemed confident that my illness was under control; she'd been told she could come with me to one of the chemotherapy sessions if she wished, but had decided it was unnecessary.

In the beginning, Bill had been afraid of my reaction to the cancer. He knew that I tended toward pessimism, a fact that we attributed to my background: I was born in London, raised while the bombs were falling, told by my parents about the murder of my grandparents and almost all my uncles, aunts and cousins by the Nazis. Bill, on the other hand, is an irrepressible optimist. We balance each other well, and it's been hard to tell over the years whose predictions have generally proved most accurate.

So Bill, a natural fighter with a strong belief in the power of the mind and a background that validated his own sense of potency in the world, had been afraid that I'd give in—mope around the house, refuse to fight the cancer.

"I don't want this to become a house of death," he'd said.

Now he was pleased with me. "I think you're handling this beautifully," he said. "Looking for information, dealing with it rationally, following the best program you can put together. ... "

We were sitting opposite each other on the porch, Bill upright in the rocking patio chair, me reclined on a comfortable wooden chaise. The breeze rustled the trembling silver poplar leaves, and a sparrow flew in and out of a wooden box we'd tacked to a nearby tree trunk, building a nest.

I savored his praise, though I seemed to be reacting no differently from the other cancer patients I was meeting on an almost weekly basis.

"I was afraid at the beginning," I told him, "that you'd despise me for being so scared. Or you'd think I wasn't fighting hard enough. Or, if I had a recurrence," and I hastily knocked on the wooden arm of my chair, "you'd think it was somehow my fault because I hadn't meditated or thought right or done all those visualizations you're supposed to or something. ... "

In fact, I now understood that you have little choice when it comes to reacting to a diagnosis of cancer, or, I imagined, to any other life-threatening event. You respond as the person you are—the product of a lifetime of actions, thoughts and decisions, big and small. If you're a happy sort, you'll swing back toward happiness again after some weeks of grieving, like one of those round-bottomed figures that simply can't be knocked over or kept supine for long. You might wish you could behave like someone other than yourself. Sometimes I yearned, for example, to exhibit Bill's quiet stoicism. But it's no good. You're stuck with yourself. You also know that weeping, yelling and snapping at friends and family might give momentary relief, but those actions simply don't touch the essential problem. "You're certainly taking all this very well," a dear friend once said to me on the phone. "There's no percentage in taking it badly," I responded. "No one's told me that being obnoxious would eliminate the cancer. If it would, I'd start snarling at you this minute."

"Look," Bill reassured me now, "I do believe that the mind has something to do with health and illness, that it can affect how our bodies behave. But to think that was the sole cause and blame you for your illness—that would be ridiculous. There are so many things—environmental factors, genetic factors—that influence our lives."

We were silent for a few minutes. Then I said, "I've been thinking about something else. If I died, would you remarry?"

"I can't think about that now. I can't think about you dying."
"But would you?"

He didn't answer. I pressed on. "I mean, I'd want you to. Really. I'd want you to be happy. And you're such a wonderful husband. All my single friends say they wish they could clone you. I'd want some other woman to have what I have now. And perhaps I could talk to Anna so she'd accept it ... "

He said, "Just think about getting well and staying well."

Through the summer, we shared many hours on that porch, rocking, talking, watching as the sparrow nestlings poked their heads through the hole in the box and chirped for food, laughing at the antics of our three dogs—one of whom, Copper, never seemed to leave my side during this period. Whenever I looked down, whether I was eating, reading or watching television, I'd find her curled up quietly at my feet.

Bill's dog, McDuff, too, was a bundle of naturally healing energy. He was the raggedy product of a match between my nervous, friendly Airedale, Petra, and an anonymous intruder who had leapt our fence one night when she was in heat. Although he wasn't fat, everything about him seemed large and round, from his huge paws (Clydesdale hooves, Bill called them) to his fleshy ears and black bulb of a nose. When he ran, his limbs seemed to wamble off in opposite directions, his hair flew out, the rough feathers of fur around his face and head rose and separated and reclustered like the petals of a disheveled dahlia.

After work, I'd walk through the gate into our tree-shaded yard, with its tangled growth of bushes, weeds and long grasses, its blossoming apple and plum trees, and watch McDuff and his mother pounding down the path to greet me. Some of the self-help books I'd read had suggested the use of affirmations: positive little sayings to be repeated to oneself several times a day, accompanied by slow, deep breaths. Now an affirmation flowed into my mind unbidden:

"The love in this house will heal me."

5
THE WALRUS AND ME

Eventually I sat down and read the book that Dr. Darcy had so hurriedly recommended when I'd sought a second opinion about surgery: Lawrence LeShan's *You Can Fight for Your Life*. I read with rising incredulity and, ultimately, fury. The book may have had some therapeutic effect in the end though: when I'd finished reading, I hurled it savagely against the bedroom wall—my first truly energetic and unambivalent act since the diagnosis.

Lawrence LeShan presents the hypothesis that there is such a thing as a cancer personality: that certain kinds of people, because of their psychological make-up, are more likely to get cancer than others. These people, briefly summarized, are melancholy, creatively blocked, unable to sustain long-term, loving relationships and apt to suppress their emotions. So if we're to believe LeShan, those of us who have cancer must bear the burden not only of the illness but of knowing that our own deficient personalities caused it.

"None of this makes any sense," I fumed to Bill. "It doesn't fit. These last fifteen years with you have been the happiest of my life. My work's creative. I love you and Anna. And as for expressing my feelings—most of my friends probably wish I'd shut up about them half the time."

Despite Dr. Fleagle's assertion that there was no known correlation, I had continued to suspect that my cancer had been caused by my seven years on the birth control pill. Although speculation is rife on this topic, the possibility of a link is always treated in the press with great caution and surrounded by disavowals. Yet the media enthusiastically tout the concept of a cancer personality, which is based on far flimsier evidence. The culpability of the pill, after all, is a serious real-world question—

and one with considerable pecuniary implications. But when you're talking about the human psyche, it seems, any half-baked, half-proven theory can gain widespread acceptance.

I also found LeShan's approach deeply offensive. He continually tossed out wild generalizations like: "Because the cancer patient has usually lost the central relationship of his life even before the development of his cancer, he feels very much alone and isolated in a hostile and uncaring universe."

His tone was that of a healthy man facing his clients with condescension and pity: "All of us, at one time or another, may be faced with a temporary situation in which we feel that no third road exists. It does, of course, but we may be unable to see it. The cancer-prone personality, however, always has that feeling: it is the fundamental aspect of his total approach to life." And: "It is often a problem to help the patient realize just how thoroughly he has rejected himself, and how much he is out of contact with his real feelings." Those willfully oblivious patients!

By contrast, the approach of Bernie Siegel, author of *Love, Medicine and Miracles*, was warmly empathetic, and I found his book comforting, even though Siegel bases much of his work on LeShan's theories.

You Can Fight for Your Life is filled with little homilies about cancer patients who recovered because they made major changes in their lives. There was, for instance, the musician (LeShan doesn't even bother to name his instrument) who had given up his dream of a concert career for something more practical. He developed a brain tumor. Feeling he had nothing to lose, he began playing with an orchestra again, and, lo and behold, the cancer receded. Simple as that, boys and girls.

The appeal of this kind of thinking is obvious. For the patient, whose sense of control has been shattered by the diagnosis, it offers hope, a blueprint to follow in the search for salvation. For a medical profession that has had little success in treating this disease, the theory offers an out: the cancer is, in some sense, the patient's own fault; on an obscure level he or she even desired it. And for those who are still healthy, LeShan's theories provide reassurance. They can believe that their own mental robustness and spiritual purity will protect them from the scourge that claims one out of three Americans.

Boulder is a community steeped in New Age thinking, and theories like LeShan's have wide acceptance here. "Just make up your mind that you want to live," I was told by several friends, "and you will." I found this deeply hurtful. It implied that I had caused the tumor in my breast through wrong-thinking or an insufficient appetite for life. It added an unthinkable volition to the death of my still-young father when I was four, to my mother's tortuous dying struggles.

It also created an insoluble dilemma. When you find out you have cancer, you are shocked, frightened and depressed. For weeks, images of death and dissolution march grimly through your mind. And then someone implies that these very sane and normal responses may in themselves prevent your recovery.

Shortly after my encounter with LeShan, I read a beautiful article by Paul Cowan in the *Village Voice* about his leukemia. It was called "In the Land of the Sick." Mindful of Norman Cousins's advice in *Anatomy of an Illness* that laughter is a healing force, Cowan had his friends rent a video machine and some comic tapes. Then he settled down to laugh himself well. Unhappily, he was in too much pain and too miserable to find the films funny. Now he was doubly damned. He had a terrible illness. And he was the kind of person who didn't deserve to recover from it.

But still ... But still ... The seductiveness of these beliefs was not lost on me. My rejection of them might be vehement, but it could not be absolute because my need was too great. In addition, while I discarded entirely the idea of a cancer personality, I knew there was mounting evidence that emotions did affect the body in complex and subtle ways. I knew that a Stanford scientist had found that women with metastatic breast cancer who attended support group sessions survived longer than women with the same disease who did not. How to pick the wheat from the chaff? Anxiously, I queried Dr. Fleagle. Had he noticed any correlation between personality and prognosis in his eight years as an oncologist? Well, he said, there was only one correlation that really seemed to hold up: "If the patient has close loving relationships," he told me, "like the relationship you obviously have with Bill, they almost always do better with the treatments. They just tolerate them better."

I called Michael Broffman, a practitioner of Chinese medicine in San Francisco, and asked him about the cancer personality.

"There might be some truth in it, Juliet," he said, "I really don't know. But I can't square it with anything I see in my practice. I can't square it with the three-year-old girl who came to me last week with leukemia. Or the ninety-year-old woman with uterine cancer I'm treating who spent last summer climbing the mountains of Tibet."

Still, despite my skepticism, I did try to think of ways in which I might have caused my cancer. Because if it was a habit of mind— or a habit of living—that had sickened me, then I could cure myself.

LeShan says that often a disastrous event of some kind has occurred in the patient's life roughly a year before the diagnosis of cancer. Cecile had died only a week before I found my lump, but we had learned she had cancer about ten months before that. And her illness and death had, of course, brought back a torrent of memories of my mother's last few months. It all seemed to fit. I presented the theory to Dr. Fleagle. "I doubt Cecile's cancer caused yours," he said. "Your tumor had been forming for two or three years." I later discovered that it can take ten years between the first mismultiplication of a cell and the discovery of a tumor.

Then there was the matter of changing your life to eliminate whatever dissonance had caused the cancer. All the literature I read urged this approach. The trouble was that I found my life deeply satisfying. My relationships with Bill and Anna were peaceful and affectionate. I loved our big, rambling house, a collection of oddly shaped spaces and passages that had begun with three dark little rooms built in the 1890s to house Boulder's first school and progressed from addition to addition—a long, narrow kitchen added in the 1920s, an airy living room constructed in the fifties—until, a few years ago, Bill topped the eastern side with a beautiful study he'd designed, all wood and windows.

As for my professional life, it was true that I had been wanting for some time to write fiction—an ambition thwarted by the long hours I put in at the newspaper. But I had been working on short stories regularly in the early morning. And I did enjoy the job: working with creative people, putting together newspaper sections that combined the talents of writers, designers, illustrators and photographers, feeding my curiosity about the world with the reams of information that flowed daily through my computer terminal. In the weeks following my diagnosis, it was the constant distraction and hubbub of the newsroom that had kept me sane. The worst days I endured were in the week following surgery, when I was confined to the house.

But I did sometimes have a sense of the things I would like to have written and had never had time for pressing against my breastbone. Was that making me sick?

I thought of other reasons, some silly, some profound. For example, I had always been faintly embarrassed by the size of my breasts. As a pre-teenager, I'd envied boys their freedom, which seemed granted by the hardness and spareness of their bodies. I'd relished my reputation at school as someone tomboyish, tough, able to wrestle boys to the ground. I lost my powers on a bright summer day, in an incident I still remembered clearly.

I used to spend my holidays at a house in West Sussex, near the little town of Steyning in England. My playmate there was a pale, skinny boy almost exactly my age, called Lesley. Each year we greeted each other with a wrestling match, and each year I won. Until the summer I turned twelve. Then I spotted Lesley coming up the path, tackled him with all my customary fervor, and within seconds found myself dumped on my backside on the ground. It seemed that over the course of the year Lesley had learned a new move. He taught it to me as soon as he had finished gloating. Even though I went on to use it quite successfully in later encounters, I associated my humiliation unequivocally with the onset of puberty.

In my teens my breasts grew large. Boys made jeering remarks about them. I saw them as a constraint, a loss of both freedom and potency. Even as an adult, I found them faintly embarrassing. When I jogged, they undulated in slow up-and-down waves, a comic counterpoint to the staccato pounding of my feet. These were the luxuriant breasts of a courtesan; they didn't suit the strong-minded, unconventional kind of woman I wanted to be at all.

Only after Anna's birth did I come fully to accept the contours of my body, the bulges, the softness. Then I gloried in my pudded-out belly because it had sheltered and protected her, loved my breasts for their ability to feed her. Potency was a word I had learned to redefine.

There were other possibilities. I had wanted to be an actress since the age of nine. When I was twelve, the head of the acting school I attended weekly in London pulled me aside to say she felt I had the requisite talent to make the stage my career. "Someday you will play Juliet," she told me. "Ophelia, Rosalind ... all the great parts." Running toward home to announce this to my mother, I literally bumped into an elderly gentleman. "I'm sorry," I said, "but my teacher just told me I should be an actress. I'm going to be an actress when I grow up."

"Really?" he said. "That's rather my line of work."

He turned out to be a retired music hall performer, a coincidence I took for a blessing on my plans. For the next half hour, we sat together on a bench while he told me stories about the theater and offered advice.

Through my teens I held fast to my goal, winning several contests around London and two scholarships for study at my acting school. But when my mother remarried and we moved to the United States, my joyous planning went awry. I attended the University of Delaware and appeared in several plays there. Then came New York. In England there had been a specific and comprehensible path: either following university or immediately after grammar school, you went to the Royal Academy of

Dramatic Art or the London Academy of Music and Dramatic Art. From there it was off to the provinces for repertory and then—if all went well—to London.

In New York there seemed to be no training standards, no tests to pass, no orderly way of getting into theater—just a kind of roiling mob of applicants (they might be people who, like me, had trained for the stage since childhood, or dentists, cabdrivers, college graduates, models, who had just decided to give acting a try) clogging the doors at auditions. I was insecure, homesick and completely at sea. Even the style of acting I'd learned seemed out of place. I struggled through, working low-paid odd jobs, taking acting classes and auditioning. Every now and then, I performed somewhere—off-off-Broadway, in summer stock, in a radio play. Eventually, I gave up.

Wracked by guilt, I conjured up other reasons. For many years I had wanted a second child. Bill and I had thought about it, discussed it, procrastinated. One night, when Anna was about three, Bill had begun making love to me unprotected. As I approached climax, I had a strong, clear vision: an infant floating toward me curled up in a fragile membrane, turning as he came, slowly and beautifully, like an astronaut in space. I thought Bill knew, as I intuited, that I must be fertile. I thought he'd decided to throw caution to the winds and make a baby. But suddenly he withdrew and began fumbling for a condom. I exploded into tears. "What is it?" he asked. "What's the matter?" I couldn't speak then, but I told him later. I had seen our unborn son moving away from us into black oblivion, and I knew he was lost to us forever.

For several reasons, we never tried for a baby again. Now I relived this incident. And I thought of a dream I'd had about two years before my diagnosis. I had seen a corpse—head back, mouth cavernous and open, long black hair turning an odd rusty color at the ends—lying in my vegetable garden. Had our denial of the son we were meant to have somehow turned my fertility into decay?

The idea of cancer as healthy growth turned destructive, the life force run amok, made sense—and it seemed especially evocative for a cancer of the breast. This idea made me fear gardening, cooking, love-making—the very activities I normally defined as life-affirming. It must mean something, I thought, that most breast cancers are discovered in May, even as the lilac blossoms, the sap runs and the birds begin building their nests.

There was one last possibility: the unassuaged guilt I felt for not having succored my mother when she was dying. Locked in absurd nursery patterns, I'd watched helplessly as all the cracks and strains in her marriage to my stepfather, all the ambivalence between her and my half-sister, returned to torment her and keep her from a peaceful death. It was as if I were underwater and struggling to surface, to intervene, while the scenes around her hospital bed came more and more to resemble hideous farce. After Cecile's death, at home, surrounded by loving friends and family members, I had envied Lynn her wisdom and ability to help her mother, her cleansing tears, her clear conscience.

The tumor had been on the inner part of my breast, close to where I imagined my heart to be, and I kept thinking of some lines from *Macbeth*: "Can'st thou not minister to a mind diseased; / Pluck from the memory a rooted sorrow; / Raze out the written troubles of the brain; / And with some sweet, oblivious antidote / Cleanse the stuffed bosom of that perilous stuff / Which weighs upon the heart?"

Perhaps fortunately, Antonio Wood had very little patience with this kind of thinking. If the unresolved issues surrounding my mother's death were still troubling me, he said, we could talk about them. But he did not believe that they had caused my cancer. "Thinking doesn't cause cancer," he said. "It's true that depression—clinical depression, which isn't something you've experienced in all this—can impair the functioning of the immune system. But all the guessing you're doing is just magical thinking. And as for the impact of mood on prognosis, in the latest study I've read, the women who survived breast cancer the longest were the worst tempered—the ones who got angriest, and were also the most hostile toward their doctors." He laughed. "I'm not quite sure what that means."

Still, he confused me sometimes, because his injunctions to stop what he called "catastrophizing" sounded so like what I was reading in the New Age books.

"Thinking about all the terrible things that can happen, picturing yourself helpless in bed, in pain, connected up to tubes, is just mind fucking," he told me. "When that happens, you can try to turn your mind to something else."

"But isn't that the same thing as Siegel and LeShan and everyone saying just be happy and think pleasant thoughts?"

It was not, I surmised later. Dr. Wood was not saying that by controlling my mind I could control my illness. He was saying that my mind was the one element in the flurry of treatments and confusion that I could keep steady and strong. And I think that, as a Buddhist and a practitioner of meditation, he also believed that working with the mind represented the highest human goal. If New Age healers recommended meditating for gain—that is, to regain health—Dr. Wood thought it should be done, if at all, as a good in itself.

Almost all the cancer self-help books talked about visualization: they claimed some patients were able to help and even cure themselves by relaxing deeply and imagining the white blood cells of their immune system battling the cancer cells. They might see these white cells as anything from cowboys in white hats to cleansing bubbles of soap. I did try to do some of these visualizations, though whether because I believed it would protect me from recurrence or simply to bring some peace and centeredness to my days I wasn't sure. But it was difficult. There were so many questions. Reading *Love, Medicine and Miracles*, I saw that it was important to visualize correctly. If you came up with the wrong image, you could do yourself harm.

What was I to imagine? If I hoped my body was cancer-free, should I be imagining cancer cells within it at all, even if they were being destroyed by whatever white creatures I chose as a metaphor for my white blood cells? Or should I just think of torrents of water pouring through my system and cleansing it? Or music bringing everything into harmony? Did you have to be able to visualize your bones, blood, organs and cells accurately or could you sort of fudge it? And what was the best creature to choose as your inner ally?

I thought of sharks—surely powerful and fast enough to snap up anything that entered their line of vision. But then, I thought, sharks are such primitive, mindless creatures. Could a shark make distinctions? Wouldn't it be as apt to tear a bloody path through my entrails as to gobble up cancer cells?

One morning, as I relaxed on the floor, an image came to me unsummoned of a beautiful white cat sitting in a window, preening. The light made pink shells of his ears, his coat was fluffed out and soft. I decided to call him Tomas and gave him a mate called Tomasina. Then I turned the two of them loose inside me. They prowled through veins and along bones, under hanging knots of muscle, in settings that I imagined as dark, dangerous and tantalizing, like the streets and alleys down by the London docks. They caught cancer cells, which I saw as large rats, killed them and dropped them into the dark whirlpool of my kidneys to be disposed of.

Although I felt great affection for the cats and enjoyed this entire scenario, it did have its drawbacks. Rats are strong, unpredictable and vicious. It isn't possible to imagine a rat-infested area being totally cleared. And cats aren't very clean killers: Tomas and Tomasina tended to play with whatever they caught so that you couldn't be sure, even when a rat was dropped, limp and wet, into the kidney whirlpool, that he was entirely dead. Furthermore, these were utterly self-willed felines. Efficient ratters when they chose to be, they were also fond of sitting in easy chairs nibbling delicately at the skin between their claws or washing their ears and faces. They slept a great deal on silken cushions. So while I retained their services simply for the pleasure of watching them, I soon decided I needed more dedicated helpers.

QuaLife, the support group that Sara Wolfe had recommended (and of which, since our phone conversation, she had become the director), held a regular visualization class. It met in

Denver every Thursday night for four weeks. I called Doris, the former breast cancer patient who had phoned the evening following my first visit to Dr. Day, and suggested we go together. She agreed.

The QuaLife office was located near Presbyterian Hospital, and, since the directions were a little confusing, we found ourselves driving up to the emergency entrance there. We parked the car and walked to the building to ask where the QuaLife office was. I was very tense, and, glancing at her as we walked together, it seemed to me Doris was, too. I think we were both afraid of seeing someone who was very sick or dying, possibly even someone in the last stages of cancer. There were things during these early months that were simply too terrifying to face, things I couldn't allow myself to know. It was almost a year, for example, before I fully realized that a breast cancer metastasis was considered incurable, even though I had doubtless been told this earlier. But we got our directions from a young nurse without incident and made our way to the meeting.

My first response to the cluster of people in the warm, shabby little office was an ignoble one. I didn't like them. I didn't want to be with them. They were all cancer patients. What was I doing there?

M. L. Frohling, the facilitator, began the meeting by having each of us introduce ourselves, and the people in the room began to assume some individuality. As it turned out, they weren't all cancer patients. There was a young woman with a bone disease that led to frequent disability and breakage; another woman was a nurse whose husband had cancer. He was in despair and refusing to leave the house, so she had come to QuaLife on his behalf. There were two breast cancer patients besides Doris and myself. One was a tall, strong young woman with long, red nails, bright, deftly defined makeup and carefully waved hair. She was the mother of two small children and held a time-consuming job, but she was determined that the cancer would not curtail her activities in the slightest. Six of her lymph nodes had been cancerous, she told the group, and her manner as she said it was almost defiant, as if she dared us to look distressed or make little noises of sympathy; she was going to be fine.

The second woman was thin, sharp-featured and intense, with curly red hair. She was, it turned out, extremely angry. Everything was upsetting to her since her cancer diagnosis, she explained at a later meeting; any minor setback could throw her into a rage.

M. L. talked a little about the immune system. To help us visualize what was going on inside us, she passed around a magnificent book of photographs by Lennart Nilsson called *The Body Victorious*. In a sequence Nilsson titled "The Kiss of Death," one of the body's protective killer cells encounters a cancer cell. By the last photograph, the latter has become a skeleton of itself: the image is of a kind of soft, blue streaming into nothingness. Then M. L. led us through some exercises designed to hone our senses and let us know our own proclivities, which of the five senses we found most evocative. She'd ask us to imagine the taste of something, lemon perhaps or honey; the sound of bells; the feel of silk against our bodies; the look of a hillside covered with daffodils. All this was immensely pleasurable. It reminded me of my old acting exercises. Only one of the participants found it useless. "I just can't seem to get any sensation," said this middle-aged woman in a flat, whiny voice. "I don't see or taste or hear anything." The speaker was, it turned out later, a five-year survivor of uterine cancer. ("If all those cancer personality pundits are right," I observed to Doris on the next car trip, "that bitter, negative woman had no business making it at all!")

M. L. turned to her assistant facilitator, Nancy Whitcomb. "Why don't you tell everyone here some of the things you've done with visualization?" she said.

Nancy was a round-limbed young woman, with pale skin and shiny black hair. Sitting silent, she'd looked a little somber. But the instant she spoke, humor and insight animated her face.

Nancy had had a brain tumor removed. After the surgery, she was told that she had a 40 percent chance of surviving. Fine, she'd thought, then I'm going to provide the remaining 60 percent myself. She'd begun exercising. As she pedaled away furiously on her stationary bicycle, she created a little song. "Oh, folks all say the tumor's gone," she sang to the tune of "Camptown Races." "They all say it's gone for good. Oh, doo-dah day." She revamped her diet. And she took up visualization with a vengeance.

Apparently, certain kinds of cancer-destroying killer cells learn their function in the thymus gland, right behind the breast-bone. Nancy saw this as a gym, populated by huge, muscular men in white T-shirts and shorts. Periodically, she would call them together and huddle with them, setting up a plan of action. Then she'd have them fan out through her body, searching for cancer cells, which they punched and kicked into oblivion.

She had other techniques. During one relaxation session, she painstakingly created a strong white, picket fence. She placed this around her brain and affixed to it a notice in large letters: "KEEP OUT. NO CANCER ALLOWED."

Nancy had twice had to undergo a brain scan called an MRI (Magnetic Resonance Imaging). Apparently, this involved lying on her back in a huge machine: "You can swallow, blink and breathe, but you can't move anything else. It's like being in a coffin." Jackhammer noises tore jagged patterns in her brain. After the first session, when the hospital staff came for her, Nancy was screaming.

By the second MRI, she knew what to expect. She relaxed her body and proceeded to work on a visualization. As the machine emitted its violent sounds, she watched a jackhammer crashing into concrete. It was pounding out a message. Slowly and deliberately, while Nancy watched every movement of the tip, making sure that each letter was perfectly and exactly formed, the jackhammer spelled out, "CANCER BE GONE."

"When I came out this time," Nancy said, "I was smiling."

The workshop became very important to me for a number of reasons. One was simply that, week by week, during the hour-long drive to and from Denver, I was coming to know Doris better. From the first phone call, I had felt tremendous gratitude toward her. After that call, she had phoned every week or so, "just to see how it's going." She would hit exactly the right tone between solicitude and lightheartedness, and the sound of her voice always calmed me. In far more detail than my surgeon had been able to provide, she had told me what the node dissection would feel like ("It isn't painful, and you can still write or play the piano or do anything that doesn't require raising your arm") and what emotions to expect.

Since we always set out right after work, with no break for dinner, Doris and I took turns bringing snacks for the trip—bagels and cream cheese, fruit, whole-wheat Fig Newton cookies. And we shared our thoughts.

"What do you think about the tall woman with the six lymph nodes?" I asked her. "Is she the healthiest person that's ever lived, or is she just denying everything?"

"I don't know," said Doris, a therapist, thoughtfully. "I suppose conventional wisdom would say she's refusing to face the cancer. But who's to say that isn't the best possible response for her?"

"Sometimes I feel really triumphant," Doris said on the way home one night. "Don't you? I mean, this is the one thing everyone is most terrified of. 'The Big C.' I've had it, and I've survived it. And I feel pretty strong for having done it."

She turned from the road to look at me—calm oval face, pretty silvery-white hair, a steady, strong gaze. I laughed, almost guiltily. I could never bring myself to say that I had survived cancer or conquered it. I subscribed to what a British novelist once described as "The Fat Man Standing by the Goldfish Pond" school of philosophy. The theory goes like this: The moment you see a fat man standing by a goldfish pond, stomach proudly protruding, hands clasped behind his back, saying in a plummy voice, "It's an odd thing, but I've never fallen into a goldfish pond," you know it'll be only a matter of seconds before some mischievous woodsprite has given him a shove, and he's thrashing around in pondscum, sputtering out great gobbets of water.

Still, I knew what Doris meant. There had been moments when I'd felt a kind of sly pride. I'd had cancer. I'd had surgery and was on chemotherapy. And, yes, I did still seem to be going strong. Most of the time, I was even happy.

Perhaps ironically, given my first reaction, one of the greatest benefits of the workshop was the simple joy and relief of being with other cancer patients. We formed a kind of community in that shabby QuaLife office, laughing at jokes no outsider would have found funny, understanding each other in a way not even the most loving spouse, parent or child could do.

One evening we had gathered in the kitchen during a break. "I have a cold," said Nancy.

"That seems so unfair," said the angry woman with the curly red hair. "It seems like when you've had cancer, you should never have to bother with minor nuisances like colds and flu again."

"Oh, I don't know," said a third woman. "I kind of like colds. You know what they are and what they're going to do. There's a beginning, a middle and an end to a cold."

"Right," said the second woman. "And they don't cut you when you have a cold."

We all began chiming in: "Or poison you with chemicals."

"Or irradiate you."

I felt a sense of easiness with my illness that I'd never felt before. "Colds are really very nice," said Doris.

Most of all, I was beginning to get more and more into the spirit of the visualizations. M. L. Frohling liked to talk about flowers, about fragrant gardens full of tea roses. Comparing her visions to Nancy Whitcomb's flat, cartoony images, I began to let go of the idea that there was just one right way to do this, and then the images came. At one point, as I relaxed, I saw myself swimming in an icy sea, stroking steadily, untroubled by cold and surrounded by the austere, shining beauty of ice floes and cliffs. All of a sudden, there was a disturbance in the water. A huge, clumsy walrus was thrashing his way toward me. His immense head was cocked to the side, his flippers sent the water spuming up around him. He positively wiggled with enthusiasm. As he came closer, I saw that it was McDuff, transmogrified. He was now a sea creature who had come to play with me. For weeks afterward I had only to look at Bill's dog, no matter how grim I was feeling, to explode into giggles.

One evening we were relaxing again into the overstuffed chairs and sofas of the QuaLife office. M. L.'s gentle voice was guiding us through a visualization. And suddenly, springing from my thymus gland, I saw Anna. She was in her white karate gi, kicking and punching with tremendous zest and concentration. She encountered a cancer cell, which was big and light and hollow, like a bubble, and burst it with one blow, laughing. Suddenly there was another identical Anna, and another and another. Dozens of them. They came tumbling out on my rushing, transparent bloodstream; some rolled in little balls, some half risen, some on their feet, feinting, jumping and hitting, eliminating the hollow cancer cells with no effort at all.

"But this is wrong," I kept telling myself. "This isn't the right image. I should be seeing the cells as stronger, the whole thing as more of a battle. And Anna is too little and light to represent killer cells. I'm doing this all wrong."

But then I realized the image was exactly right. If Anna was a delicate, small child, she was also exceptionally strong and steady in spirit. And besides, how could any image be more powerful? Anna's existence was the strongest incentive I could possibly have for living.

6
THE DARK STRANGER

I was twenty-nine and had recently moved to Boulder at my mother's urging when her cancer was discovered on a routine visit to her doctor. He held out hope that the lump he'd discovered might turn out to be a polyp, but it wasn't. Through the four years it took for the cancer to kill her, we were constantly given reasons for hope, and those hopes were constantly dashed. After the first surgery, they assured us that the tumor was small, they'd found it early, a fairly high percentage of patients survived colon cancer. There were even athletes with colostomies. But she never really recovered. Within weeks, there was a recurrence along the scar tissue. Then a second. Then all was well for a year or two, until the cancer was found elsewhere in her system, and finally in her lungs. From the first, she hated the embarrassing colostomy bag; her face never lost the strained, anxious look she'd acquired at the time of her diagnosis.

I saw her right after her first surgery. Tubes were going into her and a yellowish crust had formed at the corner of her mouth. "They got it all," we told her. "Everything's going to be fine." She nodded and made a small sound of assent.

"You may hear her moaning," her doctor told us. "But don't worry about it. She's not really in pain."

He probably meant to be kind, but his comment made me angry. My mother was one of the bravest people I knew. If she indicated that she was in pain, I knew she was.

At first she seemed to rally after surgery. I had a brief bout with flu and couldn't visit the hospital for a few days, and she sent small presents home with my stepfather, things she'd been given: a scented candle, flowers. She called and told me in her old authoritative tones to be sure and drink a lot of orange juice. I sensed that mothering me was helpful to her, allowing her to slip into an established and cherished role, reviving her spirit. I found it comforting, too.

Then they said she was ready to come home. My stepfather and I bustled about, cleaning house and preparing food. I even tied a ribbon to the collar of their little dog, Charlie, who tore it off minutes after my mother's arrival.

My mother walked through the door, looked around with a frightened, bewildered expression, sank onto the couch and began to cry. Away from the round-the-clock care provided by the hospital, she felt vulnerable and exposed. There was something else, I knew. Her marriage to my stepfather was not a happy one. Though he tended to her lovingly through the last four years of her life—feeding her and changing her colostomy bag when she became unable to care for herself—her ambivalent relationship with him was to provide an unquiet coda to a difficult life. So she returned from major surgery to a house where she had been lonely and unhappy.

My mother's great love had been my father. She had come together with him after fleeing to London at the age of thirty, as Hitler prepared his conquest of Czechoslovakia, her homeland. After she left, her mother was taken by the Nazis. My mother had often told me how it happened. It seemed that my cousin (twelve years old at the time) had been sent to stay with my grandmother in her little village. The order came for all Jews to congregate at the synagogue. Cousin Tommy had come downstairs to the kitchen that morning to find a sandwich prepared for him and a note telling him to take it and leave the village. He had gone to my grandmother's room to say goodbye but had been unable to rouse her. She had attempted suicide. Terrified, he ran off and found a doctor. The doctor was a Christian, my mother said, but a good man. "Leave her alone," he told my cousin. "Go. I'll take care of her." Clearly, he knew what was happening to the Jews and intended to let her die quietly.

But cousin Tommy had learned to trust no one. He raised a scene. I'm not sure if he called in another doctor or simply talked the first one into treating my grandmother. At any rate, she was brought back to life and taken to the concentration camp from which she never returned. Tommy, with a pair of his father's too-big boots slung over his shoulder, and clutching his sandwich, escaped, and made his way to Israel. There he became a founder of the Kibbutz movement. After the war, my mother visited him and his Israeli family once or twice. On her return she'd always laugh with pleasure and love describing him: a big, strong man with a huge handlebar mustache who, because of what he'd gone through as a boy, was afraid of nothing.

My mother also delighted in telling me the story of how she got together with my father. They'd dated once in Czechoslovakia, she said, but clearly the date hadn't taken. He had never contacted her again. On her arrival in London, she was met by a fellow Czech, who took her to a cafe frequented by Czech expatriates. "Oh," she said, seeing my father, "I know that person." Her companion called the dark young man over to the table. "Desider, this lady says she knows you."

My father looked my mother over: "I've never seen her before in my life."

But, strangers in a strange city, they began going about together. At first, each of them had a sweetheart at home. I believe my mother's first love died of some cause unrelated to the war. My father's never left Czechoslovakia. They began to fall in love with each other, and finally, they married.

Since my father died when I was four, my knowledge of this period of my mother's life came in snatches and fragments and the funny, silly anecdotes she treasured. There were certain stories I heard over and over again. How they each received a small stipend (whether from the Czech or the English government I was never quite sure) but had to report to a certain office and be available for work, generally, domestic, live-in work. My mother didn't want to find a job because it meant living away from my father. So, faced with a prospective employer, she'd pretend she barely spoke English. Asked if she cooked (as it happened, she cooked like an angel), she'd shake her head. Could she clean, then? Sorry, bad back. How about children? Did she get on with children? No, she didn't. As she described all this, she'd assume for me the expression she'd worn for these interviews, mouth stubborn and stupidly set, eyes wide, face round and impenetrable—every Englishman's stereotype of the ignorant foreigner. Finally, she said, a nice English gentleman came in. They went through the litany of question and response. "And," she said, laughing out loud, "he felt so sorry for me that he hired me. I went home and told your father, and he was furious. He said that only an idiot could have failed to fail that interview!"

My mother did work for a while as a domestic, for a family out in the country. She became quite fond of them, and they grew to love her and her exotic, continental cooking. At one point, so her story goes, she decided to make them a strudel. The dough for strudel must be pulled out over a table, until it is paper-thin. But, not knowing that such a thing existed, my mother had bought self-raising flour. Pull as she might, the pastry refused to stretch into the satiny sheet she was used to creating. Instead, it tore. But the little English children had no idea anything was wrong. They called out to their mother: "Oh, look. Come and look what the foreign lady's doing." So my mother simply rerolled the dough into a thick block, filled it with apples and baked it.

"They had guests," my mother said. She liked to tell these stories when she'd had a glass or two of wine, at one of the small tea or dinner parties we sometimes held to celebrate a birthday or the arrival of a friend from the old country. Though she was generally restrained and dignified, at these events my mother would laugh until the tears rolled down her cheeks: "They served it," she continued her story. "And it was a big triumph. They boasted to everyone about their authentic continental apple strudel."

If the English amused my mother, my father always wondered at their impenetrable national pride. "You never hear anyone boasting about how wonderful this country is," he used say, "but every banker and taxi driver believes to his bones that he lives in the finest country in the world. He knows it so deeply that it doesn't have to be said."

And my parents, too, loved England, because it offered them refuge when Jews had nowhere else to go. Many years after the war had ended, on the day King George VI died, I came home from school to find my mother in tears.

They must have been exotics in dour, wartime London, my mother and father, gay and gallant in their shabby flat, regularly feeding dozens of expatriate friends on her goulash or risotto—dishes that could always be expanded with a handful of rice, a splash more liquid.

But always in the background was the discordant music of the war in Europe and the concentration camps where their relatives were dying. Once I was safely grown, my mother confessed that when I was a baby she had often come into my room in the middle of the night to make sure I was breathing.

When I was four, my parents learned that my father's youngest sister and her husband had been killed by the Nazis. They arranged to have this sister's seven-year-old daughter, Emily, flown from Czechoslovakia to England. I was never told how they managed it. My mother spent a lot of time trying to prepare me for the arrival of a sister. She told me that Emily was older than me and would be able to tie her own shoelaces, possibly even to sew. I remained unimpressed. I wanted a brother. An older brother. "Liebling," my mother explained, "if you had a brother now, it would be a younger brother." That made no sense to me at all. "If you can bring me an older sister," I said stubbornly, "you can bring an older brother."

I was dozing one morning, seeing behind my eyelids a huge, whirling wheel of extravagant colors. "Julinci," said my mother's gentle voice, "look who's here." Standing by my mother was a big, rather plump girl, who was spouting gibberish nonstop. This much vaunted older sister didn't seem clever enough to tie her own shoelaces to me. She couldn't even speak English.

Months after Emily's arrival, my father died.

No matter how I tried in the years that followed, I could never remember exactly what he died of. I knew that he had some kind of cancer, but the specifics always slipped away. Liver, I think, or pancreas. Time and again, while she was still alive, I'd ask my mother. Time and again, she'd tell me. And with each telling I'd resolve not to forget again.

What I did know was that it wasn't the cancer that killed him. He died of a postoperative hemorrhage at six o'clock in the morning, a hemorrhage that an overworked hospital staff in war-ravaged London didn't discover in time. A childhood friend told me once, whispering urgently in my bedroom, that my father didn't have to die. It was negligence that killed him. But when I asked my mother about this, she said it was probably just as well he'd died quickly, his illness being what it was.

She had a dream the night of his death. She saw a man sitting on the rim of a volcano, arms crossed about his knees, head on his arms. She knew, without seeing his face, that it was my father. And then the volcano erupted, and the solitary figure was engulfed.

My father was involved in the war effort in some way I never really understood. At any rate, he was away a lot when I was little, and my memories of him were few, turned over and over in my mind like shiny pebbles. Those from my toddlerhood were ambivalent. I resented his absences. When my mother cried, reading his letters aloud to me, I hated him. I have a dim memory of receiving a beautiful doll by post from him and going for a walk and somehow letting that doll fall from a wall and crack her head.

The earliest image is from my infancy. I am huddled beneath a huge table with my mother and some shadowy other people. There is danger outside, an air raid. Somebody—somebody very important—is not with us. It is my father. In this hazy, dark vignette, I have somehow pulled out an eyelash. My mother comforts me, but I cry and cry.

But there were his returns. Another scene took place at kindergarten. Several little boys were yelling excitedly, "Oh, look, there's a soldier. There's a soldier." I pushed my way into the cluster of children at the window. And there was my father, striding down the street, resplendent in his uniform, come to fetch me home.

And what a homecoming. The room was full of uncles and aunts (all grownups were given these honorary titles in England, though the only ones I really accepted as family had the central European accents that spelled everything warm and comfortable to me). They were milling around a huge table, probably the very scene of my nighttime terrors. My father was revealing present after present for me and Emily: a cornucopia of Czech peasant skirts and carved ivory beads and ribbons and artificial flowers and perky little wide-rimmed hats.

When my mother called me, Emily and an adult friend together to tell us he had died, I didn't know how to react. My mother was being calm and sad and brave. Emily, whose last remnant of family he was, began sobbing immediately. I understood that crying would be the appropriate action. But I couldn't do it. Death was too big a concept for my four-year-old mind to grasp. This seemed like a mere extension of his usual absences. I was angry. How could someone as big and powerful as my daddy be kept from us against his will? I kept asking when he'd be back. Never, said my mother, never.

I went out into the garden where old Mr. Brown, the gardener, was puttering among the lupines and holly bushes. "It isn't fair," I told him. "My father's dead. And he promised to take me out shopping."

Through my childhood and teens, my father's absence made him a tantalizing figure of romance and desire, a kind of prince who would someday rescue me from a rather lonely and limited life. I had fantasies that he'd find a way of getting in touch through the mists of death. And I knew I wouldn't be afraid but would go with him trustingly and learn the secrets of the universe. I also wanted him to teach me the useful skill of becoming invisible.

So as my mother aged and thickened into an ordinary, dignified, middle-aged woman, my father remained young and slender, the enigmatic smile that in the photographs sometimes seems loving, sometimes sardonic, forever playing on his lips. He became the dark, elusive prince of all my childhood fairy tales; then Hamlet and Heathcliff and Jesus Christ; finally all the thin, tormented young men for whom I developed hopeless yearnings in my twenties.

When I was about nine, I found a cache of letters that he'd written to my mother. I was surprised to learn that he actually loved her, my everyday, bread-and-butter mother, despite the mystic bond that I had believed bound him exclusively to me. This may have been the first time I realized that I was not the only actor in this family drama and the beginning of my ability to empathize with my mother's sorrow and loss.

Through my teens, my route to grammar school took me daily past the cemetery where my father was buried. When I had time before or after school, I'd turn in at the huge, black, wrought-iron gate and thread my way through the headstones to his little oblong of earth, kept gay by my mother with geraniums. I'd weave wreaths of daisies to place by his name on the headstone, or just sit on the grass by the grave, communing with him.

A few summers before my diagnosis, I returned to London after an absence of twenty years and visited this place. As I walked through the gate, it seemed that the silence fell, like a dark cape, onto my shoulders. I crisscrossed the cemetery for some time looking for his grave, beginning to panic. Then I saw it: my name on the tombstone. Wittman. Desider Robert Wittman. A pale, cool sun illuminated headstone and plot; I could hear the dim sounds of traffic outside the cemetery's thick hedge. After all these years, I was alone with my father again.

The earth that had nourished the geraniums had been replaced by glassy, pale green stones. They looked like hard candies, covered with a soft glaze of sugar. I had a faint memory of my mother and sister arguing about this, my mother, helpless in America, not liking the change, Emily responding: "Well, if you were here and taking care of things, you could do whatever you liked. I don't have time to keep up the grave."

I hadn't thought to bring a handkerchief, and I couldn't stop crying, wiping my nose ashamedly (though there was no one to see) on the hem of my T-shirt. I fingered one of the stones. Something was thickening the air around me, though whether it was my memories or the living presence of my father I couldn't tell. At any rate, when I finally walked away from the grave, it was with a sense of some kind of reconciliation, of having acquired new knowledge. I understood then that my father was neither a saint nor a hero, but a kind and ordinary man who lived through difficult times and did his best for the people he loved. That though theirs was no fairy-tale marriage (an aunt had insisted on communicating to me her belief that my mother was a nag—and it wasn't too hard to believe!), the feeling between him and my mother had been as solid and enduring as rock, as the love between me and Bill. And my father must have felt toward me, I realized, as fiercely protective as I felt toward Anna.

After I received my own diagnosis of cancer, one last piece of the puzzle that was my father's memory fell into place. I finally knew that he was a young man full of plans for the future when his life ebbed out of him in that hospital room. That he was as alive, as filled with desire to watch his child grow up as I was now. And after years of resenting his desertion, I saw with the force of revelation how passionately unwilling he must have been to leave his fragile little family to face the loneliness of refugee living, the bleak banality of poverty, without him. And how little death respects even the hottest and most urgent desires of our flesh.

7
FAMILY PICTURES

Left alone, we were not a successful family, my mother, Emily and I. Doubtless overwhelmed by her own losses, my mother seemed unable to love this terribly needy child she'd inherited. Oh, she took good care of Emily, kept her clothed, fed and schooled, maintained an affectionate, familial tone in dealing with her, was nicer to her, in fact, on a day-by-day basis, than she was to me. But it didn't work. All three of us knew that I was the real child, the favored child. So Emily struggled continually to win the love of the only parent—indeed relative—left to her.

While Emily fought for my mother's love, I was longing—just as futilely—for hers: following her around, quoting her, imitating her in the time-honored manner of little sisters everywhere. She responded with indifference or bullying. When she spilled food on her dress or broke something, she'd tell me to confess the crime to our mother. I always did. Periodically, she hit me.

In one early memory, I'm laboring over her prized paintbox while she's in school. I have a damp cloth, and I'm cleaning the white tin between the ovals of color. As I work, I'm telling myself a little story about the most radiantly pristine paintbox in the world and my triumphant entry into Emily's affections and circle of friends. But no matter how hard I try, I can't get the box completely clean. My finger slips, a tinge of green or black or red disfigures the white tin, in rubbing it off I disturb the yellow, purple or blue. By the time Emily comes home, her paints have been worn down to almost nothing. She is not, of course, grateful for this, and she and my mother have a huge row about my ruining her things.

In movies, sorrow makes people gentle and kind. In real life, I discovered, it often causes them to flail about, blind to the pain they're causing others. I faulted my mother for her rigidity and hardheartedness with Emily, but looking back, I had to acknowledge the difficulty of being expansive and generous when your own life has fallen apart and you're wondering every day how much longer you can support your children. It was also true that Emily was a difficult child, angry and untruthful; in those days there wasn't an army of psychiatrists and psychologists about to explain that this was probably inevitable, given her history.

As for myself, I suppose that I must have contributed my share to the unhealthy dynamics of our family. It is just that I can't remember very much about it, or, indeed, about my entire childhood. What I do remember indicates a strange kind of paralysis. There was a lot of anxious watching. It seemed I could almost always understand everyone's point of view, but my understanding was irrelevant. I couldn't bring the warring parties together.

I did take action once, however—if not for the good of the family, then for my own sanity. Emily and I had been arguing. Perhaps she'd struck me, I don't remember. What I do remember was suddenly turning and advancing on her. To my astonishment, she began backing away from me, apologizing, saying she hadn't meant whatever it was that had provoked me. I came on, implacable. Once she was cornered, I realized that the top of my head came only to her chest. Still, I didn't hesitate. I bit her precisely where I reached.

She ran into the kitchen, crying. When our mother doubted her story, Emily pulled aside her apron, sweater and skirt. And there on her stomach were the two red crescents made by my teeth. It seems to me that she never hit me again.

For our holidays, Emily and I were sometimes sent to Sussex House, a home for Jewish children orphaned by the war. It was run by a superhumanly kind and efficient woman named Sophie. Somewhere around the age of ten or eleven, having gained permission to live there year-round, Emily moved out of our house. She still came to visit sometimes, on weekends or holidays.

I lived for those visits. Without Emily, our life suddenly

seemed very quiet and sad. My mother preserved our middle-class status by sheer force of will, by gritting her teeth and absolutely refusing to let us topple into poverty. She also rigidly controlled my activities. She sewed day and night, Monday through Saturday, making beautiful, one-of-a-kind dresses either for individual customers or for prestigious firms. I remember one firm in particular, Matita. I also remember her kneeling at her customers' feet, adjusting their hems, her mouth full of pins. I hated her customers for her servitude. I hated them for taking her from me. Some of these people must have been considerate and generous. Others, however, were arrogant and demanding, as were the managers at Matita. My mother was always nervous when she took her dresses in for inspection: the young men in charge sometimes sent her home to do over a perfectly good hem or move a couple of buttons. When all went well, however, and I was with her, she'd take me to a special continental shop she knew and buy us each one dark, rich piece of chocolate, wrapped in golden foil. Those were the most delicious sweets I ever tasted.

Mother started work at seven or eight in the morning and took a break at lunchtime to walk round Willesden Green buying supplies: eggs, bread, pickles, cheese, fruit. Then she continued at her sewing machine until ten at night. She might wear the same fraying coat winter after winter, but we lived in a reasonable neighborhood, and I was provided with good food, warm clothes, sensible, lace-up shoes. School, of course, was free, as were needed books, games equipment and transportation. All we had to buy was the ugly, navy blue uniform. Sunday afternoon movies were a rare treat; the purchase of a fourpenny bag of potato crisps for my school lunchbox required several minutes of calculation on my mother's part. Still, we lacked nothing of significance.

Except joy. I envied Emily, in the lively dormitories of Sussex House. I envied the poor children down the street, scrambling and yelling on the pavements. Their house had been specifically set aside by the government for single mothers, and it seemed to me we qualified. Couldn't we live there? I asked my mother. With those cheerful, noisy people? She was shocked at the very idea.

Those were not our kind of people. We were people who treasured learning. We were people who worked for a living.

When I was fifteen, I offered to leave school and go to work to help support us, but my mother would have none of it. I was her hope and her treasure, and I would have a university education (in England, at that time, only a small percentage of the population went to university). In the next couple of years, my uneasiness over our situation turned to fear. It was clear she couldn't keep up the pace of her work forever; her eyesight was already failing as a result of her hours of labor over the glistening black silks popular with her customers.

I didn't fully realize how difficult my mother's life was until many years after her death, when I interviewed a Vietnamese refugee for my newspaper. This woman supported her daughter by sewing. She, too, lived in a sparsely furnished but rigorously tidy apartment, with a sparkling little kitchen and everything stowed away in its place. I marveled at her devotion to her child, her willingness to consume her own life in work, her ability to survive in an alien culture. Listening to her heavily accented English on my tape, I came to an astonishing realization: my own mother had done the same thing. For me.

It wasn't that everything about our lives was grim. Once Emily had left the house, she and my mother were able to establish a tolerably pleasant relationship or at least to paper over their differences. They cooked together. Emily eventually took a hotel management course and astonished us with her ability to fold linen serviettes into lilies and boil live lobsters. We'd laugh and joke over dinner; then Emily and I would retire to wash the dishes. "Here," she'd say, slapping me with the dishtowel, "dry up!" As we worked, we'd sing at the tops of our voices—songs we'd learned in school about witches or blacksmiths.

Emily became engaged at the age of eighteen, to a kind, steady Jewish boy. She moved back to our house, and Alan began eating with us almost every night. It was wonderful to have a man in the house again. His family, which was comfortably off, bought Emily and Alan a pretty brick house in a pleasant suburb, and they moved in after the wedding. Alan completed his military service at a desk job and began working at one of his father's two appliances stores.

Emily was very happy. In conversation, she never called her husband "Alan," but always "my sweetheart" or "my husband" or "my Alan," with a strong emphasis on the "my." Later it was "my children, my house, my in-laws." She had finally come home.

All through my teens, my mother had been receiving letters from an Edward Erdelyi in the United States. Uncle Edward—as I learned to call him—had known my family in Czechoslovakia. It was he, in fact, who had brought Emily to us after the death of her parents. My mother told me, after they had been married for many years, that on first meeting him, she had written to my father: "Edward seems like a very nice man—but not really our type."

Uncle Edward had stayed in England until the end of the war and then left to teach electrical engineering in America. There he had married for the second time (his first wife died in a concentration camp) and divorced. In his letters he courted my mother, and, when I was seventeen, she agreed to visit him. She was very nervous in the weeks before she left, even taking to her bed with a rash and a high fever—she of the iron constitution. Finally, she went. And on that visit she married him.

It was a decision fueled by desperation. She simply couldn't continue to work as she had. And she knew he would provide the education, the stability, that she desired for me. So from the beginning, there was a terrible ambiguity about the relationship. It was a deal that filled me with guilt: Uncle Edward would take care of us financially; he would secure my future. In return, my mother would cook and clean for him, entertain his colleagues, play the role of his wife.

Before he came to London to help us pack our belongings and to accompany us on a farewell trip to the continent, I visited a Hungarian friend of my mother's and asked for instruction on how to say his name. "Air-day-yee," she told me. "Edward Air-day-yee." I practiced over and over.

Finally, I was standing on a platform with my mother, waiting for his train to arrive. As it pulled in, I saw a man whom I recognized immediately from the photographs: short, a little pudgy, with big ears, a receding hairline and a strong-featured, rather sulky face. He disembarked. "Good afternoon, Dr. Air-day-yee," I said carefully. "Welcome to England."

"Oh," he said in a pronounced Hungarian accent, looking over my head, "the luggage should be arriving. We have to check on the luggage." He charged forward into the crowd, leaving my mother and me to exchange glances and follow. Later, however, he told us that he'd been surprised by my greeting. It had been years since he'd heard his name pronounced correctly. "In America," he said, "most people call me Dr. Elderly."

He continued as he'd begun, charging through ranks of porters, arguing with taxi drivers, trying to bully Emily and Alan, who were house hunting at the time, into buying a home he'd seen and approved, loudly slurping his food, apparently unconscious of the reactions of the people around him.

He'd brought presents with him for me and Emily: two pairs of hideous red flannel pajamas he'd found on sale—the kind of garment no teenager could wear without shame.

For the dreamy, self-conscious seventeen year old I was, raised on the soft-spoken proprieties of English culture, the trip to Europe was a nightmare. Uncle Edward seemed incapable of walking. Everywhere he went, up and down cobbled streets, through glorious medieval archways, along the banks of shining lakes, on the sidewalks of major metropolises, he half stumbled, half ran, pausing periodically to gesture hugely and impatiently to my mother and me as we toiled to keep up with him. Sometimes he'd start our rented car rolling forward with one or the other of us half in it, half out. He'd barrel through crowded intersections, leaning on the horn, or go the wrong way down one-way streets. If a policeman stopped him, Uncle Edward, who spoke six languages, would completely forget the language of the country he was in. "Was ist loss?" he'd bellow to a puzzled French policeman. Or, "I'm so sorry. I understand only English" (in such a strong mid-European accent I was sure anyone could see through him) to a fat Austrian. The policeman invariably shrugged and waved him on.

His attempts to win my affection were clumsy. "Look, Julinci, see what a pretty sunset," he'd call from our hotel balcony, beaming as if he'd arranged the red glow in the sky himself. And I'd join him at the window, smiling politely, thinking that *pretty* was such a bourgeois term, so inappropriate for a sunset.

Once he stopped at a secondhand bookstore and picked out a beautiful green-and-gold bound volume of Byron's poetry. When he presented it to me, I was sincerely moved. I loved poetry, and I loved old books. But as I thanked him, he said, "You should be sure to keep this. When we get to the States, we might find out it's worth money."

His attitude toward money was understandable in someone who had lost everything and been forced, for some years, to survive on almost nothing (one of his favorite books was George Orwell's *Down and Out in Paris and London*). Still, it was peculiar, to say the least. He accumulated drawers full of useless objects. He filled his closets with things he'd bought on sale, on the assumption they'd be handy someday. He repackaged presents he'd received and sent them out to other people to whom he owed favors. If a local supermarket was selling toilet paper cheap, he'd fill our spare room with the stuff.

Mother and I were now more solvent than we'd ever been, but we lived frugally. Eating out was forbidden. Uncle Edward said that the food at home was better and cheaper. However, he suffered from a variety of physical ailments, most particularly a bad heart, and the nature of the cuisine my mother was allowed to prepare was rigidly circumscribed, becoming more and more so over time. She was not to use salt. She was to avoid fats: no butter, cheese or eggs were allowed. Cabbage, onions and garlic had to be avoided, too, because they upset my stepfather's stomach. Oh, and—a final, lordly prohibition—we were never to have lobster. In escaping from the Nazis, my stepfather had had to spend a couple of months at sea, eating little else, and had grown to hate the taste. I always thought that placing these restrictions on my mother's cooking was roughly analogous to forcing Renoir to use no more than three colors or telling Beethoven to go ahead and compose but not to touch middle C.

These dietary prohibitions were absolute: they could not be waived because we were eating at someone else's home or—on very rare occasions—at a restaurant. On the contrary, my stepfather demanded special service as the price of either his friendship or his custom.

Adjusting to life in America was difficult for both my mother and me. And the difficulties were compounded by her relationship with my stepfather. She, who had proudly supported her small family in London, was now forbidden to work. She would have been happy to be a saleslady in a department store, but Uncle Edward was a professor at the University of Delaware, and he said it was unseemly for a professor's wife to be employed. So my mother kept the house clean and entertained for him. Because of his tactlessness and insensitivity, he had few good friends, but he was eminent in his field and had colleagues around the world. Sequentially, he adopted graduate students. The young men who became my stepfather's protégés were supposed to defer to him, to run errands, to pick him up at the airport after his frequent trips abroad. In return, they would find their names on published papers and be assured of prestigious posts once they had acquired their doctorates. Of course, my stepfather felt as free to bully these students and their families as he did to bully us. He'd forbid them, for instance, to go out too often on Saturday nights, telling their startled young wives not to nag for attention. "Your husband has important work to do," he'd say. There was one factor that almost excused his intrusive conduct: he loved these boys. They were his sons.

Uncle Edward had always wanted a son—and he may have had one: back in Czechoslovakia, a childless married woman had begged him to help her conceive, and he'd obliged, he told me. He heard that she'd borne a little boy. But he never knew if this child had survived the Holocaust.

Long before his overburdened heart quietly gave out one night, three years after my mother's death, I had grown to love this fractious, restless, brilliant man. I learned to honor the principles that led to his embarrassing outbursts. In foreign affairs he was a hawk, who fumed because the Czechs had not adopted a scorched-earth policy when the Russians invaded in 1968. "Edward, they would all be dead if they had," my mother said. "Better to be dead," he'd mutter. But on the home front, he was a fierce defender of civil rights. In 1961, he asked me, with some disappointment, why I was not out demonstrating against segregation like some of my friends. A few years later, when I became a radical, his attitude was more ambivalent because of the widespread sympathy toward communism he perceived in what we used to call the Movement. "Why do you all do that gesture?" he asked, raising his fist in the power salute. "Don't you know what it means?" But then he pulled me aside and whispered, "Lenin. Now he was a great man. Everything might have been different if Lenin had lived."

When we finally became close, he told me a little of his life history. He told me how he'd been imprisoned by the Nazis, kept in solitary confinement for three months. He'd been allowed one book a week, so he always picked the fattest volume he could find, with the tiniest print. And he set up a sanity-saving system: pacing his cell at certain times of day; washing himself morning and evening to break up the long hours. At one point, his mother came to see him. "My son," she said, "whatever you've done, you don't deserve this." He treasured this moment; simply recounting her words brought tears to his eyes. But I was less impressed. I couldn't fathom the nature of a relationship in which a mother could assume guilt—of any magnitude—in a son taken by the Nazis.

Not all our exchanges were solemn. Uncle Edward loved bad puns. "What said one strawberry to the other?" he'd ask, and then gleefully yelp out the answer: "If you hadn't been so fresh, we wouldn't be in this jam." He also loved teasing me about politics. If I told him I'd eaten at a nice restaurant, "What would the comrades say?" he'd ask, shaking his head. After my marriage,

91

he insisted on buying us a washing machine and dryer. Then he'd walk slowly into the kitchen and gaze from one gleaming appliance to the other. "Bourgeois," he'd say sorrowfully. "So bourgeois."

As he aged, oddly, my stepfather became better looking. The flesh seemed to burn away, and he was transformed from a pudgy, fussy, little man into someone gaunt, soulful and dignified. He moderated some of his mannerisms, and his eyes became dark and unfathomable. Again I learned a new name for him. He was fond of English locutions, and he asked me to call him Pater. I obliged. Somewhere in the middle of those years of struggle, I had come to accept him as my father.

His relationship with my mother was, of course, far thornier, and I doubt that any outsider really understood it. There was a tremendous power struggle between them: if she followed his instructions not to work, cooked the foods he requested and was a dutiful wife, she took her revenge in a thousand angry and critical remarks. When he proposed relocating from Delaware to Colorado, she thought about leaving him. She finally had made the difficult adjustment to life in the United States. She had a small circle of friends, and she taught sewing on a volunteer basis at a local mental hospital, where the patients loved her and she was able to help some of them in the dangerous transition between the institution and the outside world. She could not bear the thought of being uprooted again. But she didn't know how she'd survive if she left Pater, either. So she came to Colorado. Something had shut down, however. She never fully took up the threads of her life again.

And yet I knew that there was some sense in which these two people loved each other. Or perhaps it wasn't love. Perhaps it was just a deep, shared understanding. They had come from the same background, they had both endured the war years and they shared the foreigner's astonishment at the odd customs and values of America. I think, too, that they needed the hurtful battle in which they were so desperately and continually locked—a battle that neither could hope to win or bear to lose.

8
A ROOTED SORROW

Soon after the colostomy, during a routine checkup, the doctor discovered the lumps around my mother's incision. They could be scar tissue, he said, but they would have to be taken out and examined.

It was nothing, my mother assured me. A very minor surgery. After it was over, she said that the lumps had indeed been scar tissue. It was when I invited Lynn and Gunner over for dinner a day or two later that I learned the truth. "Oh, for heaven's sake," said Gunner, who was in my stepfather's confidence, "is that what they told you? Well, it wasn't scar tissue. It was more cancer."

After my own diagnosis, remembering this, I couldn't look directly at Gunner. I avoided being alone with him. I was afraid that he knew some terrible truth about me, too. I felt that he shared my skepticism about the soft reassurances of our other friends and that we two alone understood that anyone with cancer was doomed. If I looked into his eyes, I thought, I'd see my own death there. "Oh, really?" said Lynn, when I eventually told her this. "You should talk to him then. When they found the lump on the side of my mother's face, he was pretty sure she was not going to make it—and he was right. But he's just as convinced that you're going to be fine. He thinks you'll just go through a bad time and then get on with your life."

Looking back after my own diagnosis, I found my ignorance about what exactly was happening to my mother odd. When I learned that I had breast cancer, I read everything on the topic I could find, soon becoming semi-expert on such minutiae as just how many affected lymph nodes generated just what statistics for survival. But my mother wanted to know nothing about her illness, and—though at the time of her first surgery, I did pull a nurse aside and bombard her with questions—by and large I, too, remained in the dark. There was just this vague sense of my mother fighting something huge, vicious and invisible. I didn't know what the recurrence along the scar tissue meant. I didn't know that there was a difference in prognosis when cancer recurs along the site of an incision and when it appears elsewhere in the body. (An appearance at a distant site is far more threatening.) And, of course, since she was trying to shield me from the reality of what was happening to her, I couldn't discuss any of this with my mother.

Over the next three years, there were other recurrences. Other surgeries. Finally, the doctors in Boulder gave up on her.

But my stepfather did not. He took her to Denver General, where a new doctor suggested that the limits of surgery had not yet been exhausted: they could intervene massively to try to save her. They couldn't be sure, however, what the quality of her life would be afterward. Pater was determined that she would have this surgery.

"He's an engineer," I said to Bill. "He thinks like an engineer. He doesn't seem at all concerned about whether her life will be worth living. Sometimes I think that if they could cut my mother's head off and keep it alive on tubes like in those horror movies, that'd be OK with him."

The night before she went to the hospital, he called us, frantic. "Your mother is being completely unreasonable," he shouted over the phone. "Please come here right away and talk to her."

She was refusing to go. She had closed the door of her room and was steadfastly ignoring the stream of visitors and phone calls Pater had stirred up in service to his cause. My knock produced only silence.

When I opened the door, I saw that she hadn't bothered with wig or scarves and her head was small, skull-like on the pillow. "I'm not going," she said, before I could speak. "I've decided." Holding fast to her decision in the face of Pater's pained meddling was absorbing all the energy the illness had left her. "I've had enough of hospitals. When I'm ready, I'll find a way to die."

She was hinting at suicide. It seemed perfectly reasonable to me. I knew she'd never really recovered from the mutilating shame of the colostomy. I knew she mourned the loss of her thick, still-dark hair. I remembered the time I had come to visit after she'd had three Adriamycin treatments. "Look," she'd said, defiant, angry, pulling off her scarf.

"It doesn't look so bad." I'd kept my tone even. "You might set a new fashion."

Now I wanted to tell her that I accepted her decision, that I was with her. But I couldn't speak. Her face was closed to me. And suddenly, without knowing how it happened, I found myself crying, my forehead against her bony, unyielding shoulder.

For long seconds, silence. Then I felt a hand in my hair, heard the gentle voice that had been with me since the beginning of time saying urgently, "Don't cry, Julinci. Don't cry." Desperately in need of comfort herself, my mother was not free to withhold comfort from me.

Instantly, the door flew open. "See what you're doing to Julie?" cried my stepfather. "See what you're doing to all of us? How can you do this, Ellushka?"

I felt like bait in a trap.

"All right," said my mother. "I'll think about it." And she turned her head away on the pillow, dismissing us all.

She was sullen in the car on the way to the hospital. There they fed her lunch while she sat, still dressed, on the edge of the bed. "This food is terrible," she told us. "You can barely swallow it. Look." And she opened her mouth to reveal a soggy block of something yellow and dissolving.

But finally, she was settled into bed. And—I don't remember exactly what led up to it—they were talking about funerals. Pater said something tentative about my father's grave in London, and suddenly she sat up. "I don't want to be buried in England," she said. "I want to be with you. I loved Desider as much as I can imagine loving anyone. But I've lived with you for the past seventeen years, and whatever we've been through, we've been through together. You're my husband. You've taken care of me. I want to be buried with you."

95

The next day, they opened her up, determined there was nothing to be done and sent her home to die.

Now Pater began thinking about sending for my sister. "There's no need for her to be here before spring," said my mother. "It'll be nicer for her then." "Oh, yes, Ellushka," he responded, "there is." She looked frightened. "Why?" she said, "Don't you think I'll l ..." She couldn't finish, struggled for a few seconds. "Don't you think I'll last until then?"

"No," he said.

Emily's arrival revivified us all. Now the mother of three large, noisy children, she thought nothing of cleaning up messes, changing colostomy bags. She spent hours in the kitchen whipping up delicacies to tempt our mother's failing appetite, running errands, massaging mother's flaccid limbs, chatting amiably with visitors.

"My Emily is taking care of me," said my mother, beaming.

Despite the moments of camaraderie in London, my relationship with Emily had remained painful and incomplete. We hadn't corresponded since America separated us, when I was seventeen and she twenty-one. I had felt that she disliked me and would prefer not to hear from me; she resented my ignoring her life, even the births of her children. But now, magically, all these problems seemed to be resolved. She was bringing joy and vitality into a sad, quiet house, just as she had in our teens.

I visited my parents one afternoon. Emily came bustling from our mother's bedroom. "I've dressed her. They're about to go for a walk." Mother had been housebound for weeks. Now she came out of the bedroom on my stepfather's arm, beaming shyly, like a bride. She wore her wig, and he helped her on with her coat. Then he leashed Charlie, and the three of them walked slowly out the door—like something out of a kid's schoolbook, I thought. Mummy and Daddy walk the dog.

"You're a miracle worker," I told Emily. She poured us each a cup of tea, smiling.

Twenty minutes later, the walkers returned. My mother took a couple of steps into the room, then leaned heavily against a chair. Her face was an odd shade of yellow, and the wig above it looked patently synthetic. She resembled, for one awful moment, a figure in a horror movie—the scene where the unquiet dead return to earth looking for the living. Then Emily jumped up, helped her off with her coat and, crooning comforting nonsense syllables, led her into the bedroom and put her to bed.

My birthday fell a week or so later, and my mother insisted that she and Emily would prepare a dinner for me. Bill and Pater sat at the table. I stood in the kitchen doorway and watched as my mother took the roast duck from the oven and shuffled with it toward the counter. Emily hovered close by. My mother took a knife to the bird, but each cut seemed to take an eternity, and between cuts she was forced to lean against the counter. I felt a rush of fury so strong and sudden that it stopped my breath. Damn my mother for pretending we could have a normal birthday party. Damn her for trying to be heroic. Damn her with her shuffling and her nerveless little stabs at the duck. My mother's arms had always been round and strong. She washed dishes so fast that I, with my dish towel, could hardly keep up; she swept through the house every Monday morning leaving all the surfaces shining. And now the flesh hung from her, and she fumbled hopelessly with the carving knife.

One night we received a frantic call. Emily and Pater were about to rush my mother to the hospital in Denver. It seemed she had started to bleed, churning red into her catheter bag. By the time we raced over to the house, everyone was gone. In the kitchen a half-thawed block of spinach dripped onto its plate on the counter.

At the hospital, the death watch began.

And instantly our cobbled-together family unity fell apart. Pater got it into his head that my mother could live if only she ingested enough nourishment. He began feeding her, dutifully, grimly, continually. She didn't want to die, but she didn't want to eat either. So she'd push the cheese or meatloaf or pudding around in her mouth, tongue it, open her mouth to show him that she hadn't swallowed. When she finally got the food down, he'd spoon in some more.

Periodically, she asked him to leave her alone, but he rarely did. It was hard enough going through what she had to, she told Emily once, without constantly seeing his hangdog face at the side of her bed.

Pater also made sure that, when he himself was unable to be at Mother's side, one of his colleagues, friends or acquaintances was in attendance. He seemed unable to hear her simple request for solitude.

Nor could Emily, who was missing her children and her home. She kept busy, spending every daytime hour by our mother's bed, straightening sheets, plumping pillows, bringing apple juice, making friends with the nurses. But she was restless. She had come to say goodbye, but six weeks had passed and our mother was refusing to die.

"Can I do anything for you, lovey?" she asked, over and over, solicitous. "No," said our mother, in tones that became progressively sharper. She wanted to be alone. She needed some silence. She had dying to do.

Eventually, my mother lapsed into silence for several days; I never could tell if this was voluntary or if she was unable to speak. Pater and Emily began talking as if they were alone in the room.

"I called my friend Esther in London," Emily said one afternoon. "It was so good to talk to her. I told her to look in on Alan and the children. And then she asked about Mummy. I told her, if I ever get like that, just shoot me."

Several minutes went by. Emily had moved on to another topic. Suddenly my mother's blurred, cracked voice came from the bed. "Why don't you go home?"

"Oh, no, lovey," said Emily immediately. "It's only two o'clock. I don't need to catch the bus home till five."

Once, she and I were walking down a corridor with two of the nurses. "It was just impossible trying to wash the old lady today," said one. She was talking about my mother. "Yeah," said the other laughing, "she was so slippery. She was just like a big old slippery piece of bacon." I was furious, but Emily was laughing. I realized that this must be the way nurses talk among themselves—

and that, since she didn't mind it, they had included my gregarious sister in their circle.

The hospital's routine assaults on my mother's dignity did nothing to ease her dying. Being called by her first name by nurses and doctors half her age troubled her. At night she still tried continually to get up from her bed and go to the bathroom. Even though she had a catheter and couldn't urinate, she had told us that simply being able to empty the bag gave her a kind of emotional relief. But one night at the hospital, she fell unnoticed and struggled on the floor, perhaps for a long time. From then on, she was pinioned to her bed to sleep. I understood the need for this. The hospital could hardly station someone in her room every night. But I ached for her. To have gone through so much and now to spend her last days being treated as an object, given too little painkiller as was customary in those puritanical days, shunned by her doctor, who had clearly written her off.

Could she have gone home to die? No, said the doctors. She'd have needed a special bed and equipment and somebody in attendance who was trained to take care of her. There was no hospice movement then, no support for this kind of decision.

I seemed to have been locked into my customary paralysis. I simply couldn't break through the frantic and continual carousel of activity revolving around her bed and help my mother. Periodically, I tried. "You know, I've read that even when people seem unconscious, they often hear what you say," I said to Emily in the elevator an hour or two after her remark that she'd want to be shot if she were ever in our mother's straits. "So I think we should be more careful what we say in front of her."

"Oh, I know that," she said. "I always am careful."

I did try to give my mother some silence. Periodically, Bill would inveigle Emily and Pater out of the room for a cup of coffee, so that she and I could be alone. The tension would ebb from the room.

In the weeks before Emily's visit, my mother and I had made some progress in resolving our own vexed relationship. Somehow, even during her illness, I had been unable to shake an old fear that my powerful mother would completely dominate me, would obliterate my very essence. There was a childish part of me that almost saw her sickness as a ruse, a maneuver to draw me in and hold me, choking, to her breast, forever. I had fought so long and hard for my independence. But in the long, sad months of her decline, I had finally come to understand that while mentally I stood, fists at the ready, in the ludicrous position of a boxer who has just heard the starting bell, my mother had long since stopped fighting. At some point, unnoticed by me, she had simply dropped her hands to her sides. I will love you as you are, she had said silently. I will be your dear, dear friend.

I had finally heard her; there had been some peace between us. We talked about her life, about my marriage to Bill, whom she adored. But all serenity was shattered soon after Emily's arrival, and every stupid rivalry, every unresolved issue among the three of us came back into play. The problems between Pater and my mother, of course, had never diminished. The family interplay was like an exemplary tale or some smug, self-righteous religious text: every lapse in love, every necessary word left unsaid, every accusation hurled in anger was coming back to haunt my mother, to keep her from an easy death. A sonorous phrase from the Bible kept marching through my thoughts: "God is not mocked. As a man sows, so shall he reap."

Now, alone with my mother for a few minutes, I sat by her bed. Slowly the sense of peace and reconciliation returned. I thought about how I'd praised her singing when I was a child and how I'd compared her white, slender hands to those of Queen Elizabeth I in the old portraits. I mulled over what I'd heard about her life in Czechoslovakia. She used to tell me that she was plain as a young girl, while her sister, Ida, had been the town beauty— so beautiful that her name was known as far away as Prague, and hopeful suitors had paid the gypsies, night after night, to play beneath the sisters' window.

But in the old pictures, I was thinking, my aunt is stern and expressionless, while my mother has the sweet, secretive smile of the young Vivien Leigh.

A sound startled me. My mother's hand was fumbling at the bars at the side of the bed, looking for a space, finally beating against them urgently, like the wing of a trapped bird. The hand was seeking mine, I realized. The queen summoned. I took it.

One morning we came in to find her sitting up, alert and able to speak. "So there you are," she cried joyfully as we walked into the room. "I was waiting for you." She tried to smile, but her mouth was so dry that her upper lip didn't slide back down. It stayed suspended, stuck to her gum in what looked like a snarl.

There was a lot she wanted to tell us. It was hard to make everything out. But then she said quite clearly, "I'm glad." She rolled her head from side to side on the pillow: "I'm glad. I'm glad. I'm glad. I'm glad."

What was she glad about? That we had come? That despite everything, despite our crazed and fractured web of relationship we were all together? Or was she glad that she was dying, that it was almost over?

"My father came to see me last night," she said, a little later. "He stood right by the bed and asked how I was doing."

"No, Ellushka," Pater said, before I could stop him. "Your father is dead. He has been dead for many years. You must have been dreaming."

"Tell me about it," I broke in. "Tell me about your father."

But my mother closed her eyes. "I must have been dreaming," she said.

The burst of joy subsided, but my mother continued to speak. Against all expectation, she had rallied. Now no one knew what to do or what to predict, and day followed day with no resolution. One afternoon an intern came in with transfusion equipment: my mother had become dehydrated, he explained. Emily interposed herself between him and the emaciated figure on the bed. "Leave her alone," she shouted. "She doesn't need this. Can't you leave her alone with all your medicines and needles and operations?" But Pater pulled Emily aside and told the bewildered young man to proceed.

"Can't you see she wants to die?" said Emily, crying in the corridor.

"No," Pater said. "She doesn't."

"I heard her all the time when she was still at home. Every night. She said, 'Oh, God, please take me. Oh, God, why don't you take me?' You heard her, too."

He gave a wry, resigned little shrug. "You don't understand," he said. "She doesn't mean it. With us, it's nothing. It's a figure of speech with us."

And here was the odd thing. Though I sometimes shared Emily's feverish desire to see an end to our mother's suffering, coupled—oh how guiltily—with a longing to be freed of the burden of this long dying, I knew Pater was right. It was clear that my mother was still fighting for her life.

Nobody informed us, as hospice workers do today, how to tell when the end is near. I went on living in a kind of suspended animation, moment to moment, expecting neither death nor recovery. One evening, sitting beside my mother, I noticed how labored and audible her breath had become. Periodically, it seemed to leave her body, to rattle off into the air. There'd be a moment of white, blinding silence. Then she'd take her breath back to her and begin again.

The next day, before any of us arrived at the hospital, she died quietly, while the nurses were washing her face.

I had a dream a year or so later. My Aunt Ida was dying. The people tending to her were clumsy, inattentive. I was screaming in a fury. "You've got to do this right. You've got to figure it out. Do you want another botched death on your conscience?"

But perhaps my mother's death wasn't entirely botched. It did seem that in the last few days her soul slipped into a gentle and quiet place. I remember one of her last clear sentences. It was noon. She was gazing out of her huge picture window toward the mountains as a brilliant Colorado sun illuminated the room.

"You'd better go home, my darlings," she'd said to us—so tenderly. "It's getting dark."

9
THE OLD ONES

I knew I was lucky not to have lost my breast, and later I came to appreciate this. At first, however, I almost envied the women I knew who had had mastectomies, even double mastectomies. I thought they were safe. My breasts were dangerous. They could harbor my death. At times I wished I'd had the courage to have them cut off.

There are women whose response to breast cancer is to examine their breasts (or the one breast remaining to them) obsessively, over and over again. "I'm doing well when I get it down to eight times a day," one friend told me. My reaction was different. I wouldn't touch my breasts. They seemed alien, as if I had them on loan. I was afraid of my entire body. Sometimes my fingers would brush against a perfectly ordinary knot of flesh or protuberance of bone, and I'd feel a moment's panic: has this knob on my wrist always been there? Is there a similar knob on the other side? Or my tongue would encounter a rough spot or a tag of skin on the inside of my cheek, and again there'd be an instant of shock. Is that OK? Could it change into anything dangerous?

We'd been fairly casual about nudity around our house. We customarily slept naked, took brief trips from the bedroom to the kitchen or bathroom unclothed. Now I found that when I stripped off my clothes at night, my teeth would begin the uncontrollable chattering I'd first heard lying on the gurney, right before surgery. I began wearing an old blue-and-white striped robe of Bill's around the house and even slept in it. After a few weeks, I challenged myself to sleep naked again. Then I'd get into bed and simultaneously wiggle the robe off and pull the covers up to my collarbone as I settled down to read.

Taking a bath, or later, after the incision had healed, a shower, was an instant reminder of my mortality. This was where I'd rediscovered the tumor. I'd hold the bar of soap between the palm of my hand and the skin of my breasts and, as I soaped, keep my eyes fixed on the evergreen branches waving outside the window. Then I'd dry off rapidly and, bra safely clasped and breasts covered, heave a brief sigh of relief. Another morning. Another ablution. No new lump.

I felt that my body had betrayed my trust. I had always taken reasonably good care of it; in turn it had functioned easily and well. During my pregnancy, I had been amazed at its efficiency. Overnight, it seemed, I lost my appetite for coffee and chocolate and discovered a strong and appropriate craving for eggs, milk and vegetables. If I went too long without eating, I trembled with hunger.

I remembered my obstetrician talking to me about weight gain. He leaned forward solemnly, hands clasped on the desk in front of him. "You should gain twenty-five to thirty pounds," he said. "We now feel that that's optimum. We used to tell women to gain no more than fifteen."

I wanted to laugh at the impudence, the intrusiveness, of this man. "I'm sure," I said, as politely as possible, "that my body will gain what's necessary. By the way"—a tad less politely—"how did you ever explain you were wrong to all those women with underweight babies?"

I argued, too, about the enema routinely administered before the birth. This is a very uncomfortable and humiliating procedure for a woman enduring the violent cramping of labor. I understood, I told the doctor, that in preparation for birth, one's body simply voided all waste. Couldn't I do without the enema? No, he said, that wasn't wise. However, the day preceding Anna's birth found me making several trips to the bathroom—my assumption had been correct. And, fortunately, my labor progressed so fast that by the time I reached the hospital an enema was out of the question.

The moment of Anna's birth found me awake, undrugged and ecstatic. I was filled with a blissful sense of potency. The knowledge of how to give birth had, as I suspected, been locked in my tissues.

And my body knew how to feed the baby. "My breast milk seems to vary," I told Anna's pediatrician a few months later. "Sometimes it's kind of thin and blue, sometimes more creamy-looking. Is that possible?"

"Yes, indeed," he responded. "Breast milk changes as the baby grows. It even changes slightly when she's ill, to provide for her new nutritional demands. It's amazing stuff."

Now this body, with its miraculous knowledge of how to form and nourish a baby, had created a cancer. Secretly. Some cell had moved out of control, had been permitted to survive and double—over and over again. Then my body had sheltered and nourished the monstrous growth for what may have been as long as ten years until finally, on a sunny morning in May, it had insinuated itself as a palpable lump against my fingers.

Many years earlier, Bill, too, had felt his life threatened. He had been running along the Boulder Mall with Anna, then two years old, on his shoulders, me running behind them, and he had felt a breathlessness, a heaviness in his chest, a pain radiating outward. He didn't mention it immediately. We got into the car, and I began driving home. Suddenly, he told me to turn around and drive to the hospital. Once there, he became the center of a flurry of activity. He was hustled into a bed, his body hooked up to tubes. A mild heart attack, said the doctors some time later.

A battery of tests taken in Denver, however, showed no damage to the heart muscle, and the doctor there cast doubt on the Boulder doctors' diagnosis. But for weeks afterward—at work, eating in a restaurant, washing dishes—Bill would suddenly feel his heart fibrillating. I'd see his hand go to his chest, the fear in his eyes.

The episode, as we began calling it, led Bill to make a series of deliberate changes in his life—not all at once, but year by year. One of these was a decision he'd made, six months before my diagnosis, to leave his job as head of the advanced planning department at Jefferson County by August and become a private consultant. We decided he should stick to this decision despite my cancer.

"It's something you need to do," I said. "I can tell how bone-weary you are of the place. And even though I fantasize about

105

leaving the newspaper and writing full-time, I still really enjoy working there. So I can stick it out for a while."

Drawing on his own experience, Bill tried to guide me through some of the emotional ups and downs I was feeling.

"There was all this ecstasy mixed with the fear at the beginning," I said. "But now it's all different. I'm upset and angry and scared, and that sense of being really awake that Dr. Wood talked about is gone."

"It's not a bad thing when you finally understand that you're mortal, Bear," he'd tell me gently. "There's this monumental change at first. All this emotion and that feeling that everything in life is very precious to you. And then things return to normal. But they don't completely. You enter a new phase where subtle changes keep occurring. In the end you become a different person."

For the moment, however, my strongest emotion remained anger. The day I returned to work after the surgery, I picked up the latest issue of the newspaper's Sunday magazine, which I generally edit. I saw that a story I had assigned on eating disorders had been completed, edited and printed. It began with an interview with a woman who had filled gelatin capsules with lye and swallowed them, intending to destroy her stomach. She was slowly recovering. Normally, I would have felt pity, if not empathy, for such a person. Now I found myself shaking with anger. This woman—this blind, self-involved fool—had deliberately attacked her own God-given body, had chosen to poison it with caustic chemicals. And she was probably going to be just fine. While I, who had always treated my body with care and affection, was stricken—through no volition of my own—with cancer. And now she was asking for pity. It was monstrous.

I found other targets for my fury. Soon after surgery, the tube still hanging from my armpit, I'd gone to Alfalfa's, Boulder's health food supermarket. I was pleased to find myself able once more to engage in an ordinary activity like shopping. But I was also wondering if the miasma of sadness and fear I breathed was going to be permanent. Studying the shelves of books, I found that all the books about cancer were in the upper right-hand corner—

far beyond the reach of my poor unable-to-straighten right arm. I found the resident herbalist and informed her of this. "No one who's had any kind of surgery is going to be able to reach those cancer books," I told her snappily. "I'll look into it," she said.

I wheeled my cart to the cash register. A muscular young man in shorts and sandals was standing just ahead of me with his cart. "Hey," he yelled across me to a pretty, dark-haired woman, "Haven't seen you in ages. How ya doin'?"

She walked toward him. "Terrible." Her mouth turned down like a clown's; her voice was a wail. "Everything's a mess. I didn't get any of the courses I wanted, and I've got this horrible history professor, and my mom's still nagging me about what I should major in, and ..."

I wanted to take three swift steps across the store and slap her. Hard. "You don't know terrible," I wanted to scream at her. "You don't know the meaning of terrible."

My entire world view had changed. I was afraid to read obituaries. The death of anyone around my own age seemed like a direct threat. I noted all the clichés: "after a long struggle with cancer," "having battled cancer for several years." In the American media, it seemed to me, all metaphors that didn't relate to sports related to war. But I didn't feel I was fighting a battle. I seemed more to be gathering things together—Dr. Wood's fragments of wisdom; skilled medical care; the loving concern of friends; the sight of my daughter; Bill's steady, warm affection; our family's bright summer days and tender nights—and spinning them into a fine, soft blanket, a consolation and a magical source of strength and health.

Previously, when I'd seen a very old man or woman walking shakily down the street, I had felt pity. I had tried to imagine how it felt to know that one has only a few dimming months or years left on this sweet earth. Now what I felt was envy. I knew that I might not be given the number of years that septuagenarian had already enjoyed.

Still, there was comfort in old people, an oblique sense that if anyone was permitted a long life—if such a thing were possible—

I might survive into old age, too. When I saw an obituary for a ninety-nine-year-old Gertrude, Lurlene or Elbert in the newspaper, I wanted to sing hosannas. I felt that their longevity was a victory for the entire human race. I wanted to talk to old people, and read their books, and drink in the wisdom of their accumulated years.

In this spirit, I revisited two octogenarians, the two great heroes and teachers of my adolescence—Laurence Olivier and Graham Greene.

I learned that Greene had just published a new novel, *The Captain and the Enemy*, and I excitedly called the publicist at Viking to order a copy. Although this book was slighter than Greene's fullest and most realized work—*The Power and the Glory*, *The Heart of the Matter*, *The End of the Affair*—I saw that in it he was still struggling with the same themes: What is God? What is the nature of virtue, even saintliness? What is the meaning of human love? And, poor, weak creatures that we are, how can we escape betraying these things?

I thought of a scene in one of the first Graham Greene novels I'd ever read, *Brighton Rock*. The main character, a petty criminal called Pinkie, is fleeing razor-wielding enemies. A lapsed Catholic, Pinkie has always believed he can save his soul by repenting in the moments before death. As he runs, he fumbles desperately for a prayer. Nothing comes. The ability to pray, he realizes with overwhelming despair, is the result of habit. Salvation does not come in a brilliant flash of light, but from years of humble effort.

I knew Pinkie was right, too: a life is made up of a chain of habits, of daily choices. Whether you walk the dog or sit by the television, caress your child or curse her, read of foreign affairs or romance, cook or eat out, the fabric of your life is woven of these insignificant decisions, and you cannot go back at the end and unstitch the weave. But sometimes a very small change in the way you put the stitches together can ultimately reshape the entire pattern.

After *The Captain and the Enemy*, I took up Anthony Holden's biography of Laurence Olivier. I had loved the actor since the day my mother dropped me off at the age of twelve at a cinema where *Wuthering Heights* was playing and gone off to do her shopping. As I walked down the carpeted aisle, an earlier showing of the film was just ending. A man with tormented eyes held a dead woman in his arms. He was pleading with her to return, to haunt him, to drive him mad—but not leave him in a world she had abandoned. "I cannot live without my life," he said hoarsely. "I cannot die without my soul."

From that moment, I was ruined for the skinny English boys who kissed me tentatively in doorways. The image of Heathcliff/Olivier fused with that of my lost father, became the unattainable ideal, a passion like his and Cathy's—dark, stormy, doomed—the very definition of love. I barely breathed as the film began again and I watched it through: the dialogue that seemed illumined by flashes of lightning; Heathcliff's smoldering, damped-down fire as he was forced to perform servile chores; Cathy's confession to her servant, Nelly, that she and Heathcliff shared one soul.

That was the beginning of my one-sided love affair with Laurence Olivier, but it wasn't the end. Consider his arrogant, aristocratic Darcy in *Pride and Prejudice*, his robustly charismatic Henry V, the way he handled the black mask and lace cravat of the highwayman Macheath in *The Beggar's Opera*. Consider, above all these, his malign black snake of a Richard III, mesmerizing poor Lady Anne with a combination of lyrical poetry and willful authority, so seductive in his absolute evil that he forced the audience to empathize with his every hideous scheme and bloody murder.

This was not just a springtime romance. As I grew older, I was able to appreciate Olivier's judgments as an artist, his daring choices, the elegance and subtlety of his phrasing. When he began playing middle-aged characters, his profound sexuality was subsumed in astonishing and vital eccentricities, juicy character quirks. I remembered him especially as Archie Rice in John Osborne's *The Entertainer*, soft-shoeing his way across the apron of the stage, begging for laughter and approval and petulant when he failed to get it, singing in a cracked tenor, "Oh, ain't you glad you're normal?"

109

In the last years of Olivier's life, the accumulated effects of his many illnesses prevented him from acting on stage. But surely, I thought, the creator of so rich a gallery of characters, an artist so fulfilled, vigorous and admired, must be able to face the prospect of his own death with equanimity.

A year or two before my cancer diagnosis, I had seen Olivier on television, trudging ill-humoredly toward death as the elder Mortimer in John Mortimer's autobiographical *Voyage Round My Father*. Asked why he was so irritable, the character responded, "I'm always angry when I'm dying."

Olivier must have known that he was not too far from death himself when he took on that role, might almost have been rehearsing for it. Surely that meant he had fully accepted his own mortality. Besides, I saw a kind of shining in him as he lay on his fictive deathbed, a gentleness and steadiness that bespoke a man who had looked into the darkness and seen the light beyond.

But according to Anthony Holden, when asked how it felt to know that his work would be admired for centuries to come, Olivier responded tartly: "It is just as cold in Westminster Abbey as it is in the village churchyard. I don't want to die."

As I visited these old friends, my chemotherapy continued. One morning, I was shaking a white-blue Cytoxan tablet from the bottle when it fell into McDuff's dish on the floor. I considered briefly whether anything in the dog's saliva or his leftover food could possibly be as noxious as the chemicals in the pill, then wiped it off and swallowed it.

Dr. Fleagle had prescribed Xanax to take the edge off my anxiety on the mornings preceding treatments. But one Wednesday, I found myself drifting into sleep at the wheel of my car as I navigated toward work. Frightened, I fought the sleepiness. A few minutes later, my car scraped jarringly along the center divider on Broadway. By the time I reached work, I had decided never to take Xanax again. "It's not as if it really does anything for the fear," I told Bill later. "If anything, it seems to make me more jittery and anxious on chemo days."

Gunner had some time off from his cab-driving job, and he and Lynn decided to take Anna to the mountains for a week of camping with their daughter Dana. It was a great relief to me to have her out of the house. I still found it difficult to face her. She was such an insightful child, I was sure she could see the fear that periodically overcame me.

On their return, Lynn called me up.

"I think you should know about a conversation I had with Anna," she said. "We all went out one afternoon to see a bat cave—just a huge hole in the ground, but it frightened Anna. Next day, Gunner and Dana went off somewhere, and Anna and I were together in the hot pool. She told me she'd had a dream. She dreamed that our dog Abby fell into the bat cave. Dana had her on the leash, so she fell in, too. I grabbed Dana, but couldn't hold her, and Gunner grabbed me. We were all falling. Anna said, 'I had to catch hold and save all of you. And then I had to go through the rest of my life with my arms like this.' And she held out her little arms in front of her, stiff as boards."

"Was she joking? Did she smile?"

"No," said Lynn, "she was deadly serious. You know," she went on, "children often feel they're responsible for the things that happen in their families. Especially children Anna's age. It's an age when there's a lot of magical thinking. You might try talking to her."

A few days later, Anna and I did talk. She didn't respond at first when I asked if she felt my illness had anything to do with her, but I could tell she was listening closely.

"You know when you have a headache?" I said. "I always feel terrible. I try to bring you medicine and wet washcloths and make it better. And you've said that sometimes just having me around makes it easier to handle. But I can't make it go away. I can't stop the pain.

"And you can't control what happens to me. Whether I stay well now—which I certainly intend to do—or not. If I get kind of sick around the chemotherapy and throw up. But having you and Daddy in my life helps me get through these things. Do you know what I mean?"

"Well," she said, "when I'm at a sleepover and I'm afraid of the dark, sometimes it helps to know that Dana's in the room with me. Even if she doesn't talk, I'm glad she's there."

I blessed her capacity for understanding. "Yes," I said. "That's exactly it. That's what you and Daddy do for me."

On and off, I thought about visiting a massage therapist. My family had been interested in shiatsu massage and Oriental medicine in general for some years. It began when Bill was searching for relief from his devastating cluster headaches. These are a kind of migraine, shorter in duration (Bill's lasted anywhere from ten minutes to four hours) but far more painful. Sufferers generally get one or several a day over a discrete period of time. Then the headaches disappear for months or years.

Bill had seen several doctors and had even had a CAT scan. He'd been given drugs. But the Ergotamine the doctor prescribed had frightening side effects, and Sansert, another drug, seemed to decrease the intensity of the headaches while increasing their frequency and unpredictability. On the advice of a friend, Bill had visited a massage therapist, Jim Cleaver.

He was delighted with the massages and began talking about meridians and pressure points and energy flow. I thought he was crazy. But then Jim referred him to acupuncturist Bob Flaws, and, miraculously, through a combination of herbs and acupuncture, Flaws banished the terrible headaches. They didn't leave immediately, of course. It took a week or two for the cluster to come to an end, so that the first time we questioned whether it was, in fact, Flaws's ministrations that had stopped the headaches or whether Bill had simply come to the end of his cycle. But Bob continued to repeat the miracle, year after year. And, most persuasive proof of all, if a headache did slip through, Bob could actually stop the pain on the spot with his needles.

Meanwhile, hoping to stay relaxed and avert future headaches, Bill was still visiting Jim Cleaver. He came home from these sessions ecstatic. "You really should see Jim," he'd tell me, with an irritatingly cherubic grin. "This guy has the most wonderful hands. You wouldn't believe what he can do with his hands."

Finally, I became curious enough to visit the little white room where Cleaver plied his trade. I was met by a slender man with long, black hair. I was not impressed. Cleaver had me take off all my clothes except for a T-shirt and underpants and lie face down on a mattress. I inhaled the fresh smell of laundry soap.

Then Jim began working on me, massaging from my shoulders down to my feet. Each specific point he pressed called an answer from my body: a kind of electrical tingle sometimes, sometimes something deeper, like the vibration of a massive bass chord. Many of the spots also seemed to have some emotion or memory to yield—as if certain events had become caught in my flesh, and Cleaver were releasing them. The images behind my eyelids, as he worked my back, were a kind of solemn blue-black purple. From my left side, just above the hip, emanated a crystal clear vision of myself as a child, out shopping with my mother on a winter's day, Christmas lights shining on rain-wet streets.

Later, I couldn't remember all the things Jim did. I remembered him raising little pinches of the tight skin along my spine and twisting them ("You have a wonderful future as a mother cat," I told him); picking up my legs by the ankles and moving them; taking a hand by the wrist and shaking it to and fro as if I were waving at him (a move I found hysterically funny); paddling with his hands in my stomach.

I felt as if my limbs had been dead, and Jim, godlike, was working life into them. He took up a hand, and a photograph I'd seen flashed into my mind: it showed a dead man, a victim of the Salvadoran death squads, his head and hands being kissed by his grieving wife and children. I started to cry. That such terrible things happened in the world. That so much gentleness and love should be lavished on a body that had been treated so cruelly in life. Yet it also seemed that what was emanating from Jim's hands was a kind of universal tenderness, a forgiveness so pure and profound that it could heal the hurts of the world.

Then everything changed. I was flying up, up, out of an icy crevasse, gleaming chasms of ice all around me, into the pure, bright light of the sky. I never could find words for what happened next, only metaphors. But I found myself weeping for joy. "It was as if the heavens had opened," I told Bill later, "and all the angels were singing, 'Holy, holy, holy.'"

113

Suddenly, the light was gone. I lay in absolute darkness, filled with a profound sense of peace. Jim Cleaver had placed his cool hands over my eyes.

I was embarrassed as I dressed. I thought of massage as a self-indulgent pastime of the very rich, not the stimulus for some kind of religious ecstasy. But I couldn't deny the power of what had happened to me, or how fervently I longed, in the years that followed, to re-experience that explosion of joy and certainty. Because it was never repeated during subsequent massages, no matter how generally delightful I found them.

Before I saw Jim, I had had a dream. I was in my old acting class in New York, and the teacher was selecting students for an improvisation. I was ravenous to get up on stage, and I waved my hand frantically in the air, vying with all my might for his attention. But he finished the selection without calling on me. On my return home, I saw that the piano in our living room was cracked from top to bottom.

These were obvious images. Clearly, I felt creatively stifled. But after that first massage, I got into a play. I also enrolled in a writing class and promptly wrote three short stories. Jim had talked about how small, subtle things can have huge impacts, and certainly it seemed that his low-key ministrations had done wonders for me. When I thought of the action of his hands on my body, I'd see an image of ice cracking on a winter-locked river, the warm waters starting to flow again. To his great credit, Bill listened to my ecstatic babbling about all this without gloating.

We were now thoroughly hooked on the benefits of massage. When Jim left town, I visited one of his students, Inch Bacon. When she, in turn, departed, she recommended a student of her own: tall, beautiful Christa Forsythe, whose combination of strength and delicacy in massage stemmed from her long training as a dancer.

There was something that moved me deeply in the work of these massage therapists. The generosity, the humility of it. To kneel beside another human being, as they did, freely giving their skilled and caring touch, placing their fingers without revulsion in the whorls of their clients' ears, tugging on our little toes. Inch and Christa attended births, working to control pain, helping the baby to come. They volunteered for hospice, too, laying their hands on the dying—who are so often starved of touch. And since massage was part of what they defined as their spiritual practice, these therapists charged their clients very little, far less than a regular therapist charges for simply listening and talking.

After my surgery, I longed to see Christa. But my body was still shrinking from touch. I was also unsure whether massage would be good for me; its purpose, after all, was to unblock energy, to get things flowing, and it seemed that perhaps for cancer patients, the less flow the better. "It'll be fine," said a Chinese doctor I consulted, "as long as she stays away from the area where your tumor was."

I waited for three or four weeks before driving to Christa's mountain home and lying down on her mattress, reflexively covering my breasts with the snow-white blanket she provided. She began working on me, very gently. Deep massage could come later, when I was stronger. She was making the odd, tender little humming sound in the back of her throat that came from her at her most concentrated. I wept at her touch, but wherever she placed her hands, my body seemed to relax and soften. I was thinking of how this mild discipline of fingers differed from standard medical practice. I thought about surgeon John Day standing by my unconscious body, cutting it open with a knife. And then a comforting thought slipped in. Perhaps, I thought, John Day wielded his scalpel with the same exquisite tenderness and care that I felt in Christa's hands.

At our next session, I relayed this idea to Dr. Wood. "He does," he said. "That's how a surgeon does his work."

Eventually I would witness this for myself.

10
ANCIENT HEALING

Shortly after my diagnosis, I called a colleague of Bob Flaws's in San Francisco, Michael Broffman. The attitude of my Western doctors toward my interest in Chinese medicine varied. John Fleagle was clearly skeptical. Practicing in Boulder, he must have been aware that many of his patients were experimenting with alternative therapies in addition to the drugs he gave them—from mistletoe extract and blue-green algae to such relatively uncontroversial approaches as ingesting large amounts of beta-carotene. He said nothing to discourage me, only giving me a couple of warnings. I should be sure that I knew what was in any capsules I was given, he said. And he also wanted me to be aware that one of his patients, who was following a macrobiotic diet (this is not based on centuries-old tradition, as is Chinese medicine, but is the invention of a Japanese man named Michio Kushi), had been admitted to the hospital suffering from malnourishment.

By contrast, surgeon John Day was very interested in alternative therapies and often asked me what my Chinese doctors were saying.

Broffman responded to my query immediately with a long letter in fine, spidery writing, detailing dietary and lifestyle instructions. He enclosed an extensive list, compiled by Patrick M. McGrady, Jr., of Canhelp in Washington, of different kinds of cancer treatments being offered all over the world: in Canada, in Germany, in various parts of America. They ranged from hyper-aggressive use of conventional chemotherapies to prescriptions of what I came to call the "garlic and apricot pit" school. Although this flood of information was confusing, it did alert me to the breadth and complexity of available treatments, and it served as some reassurance that, should I suffer a recurrence despite Day, Fleagle and Aarestad's ministrations, there were still options I could follow. At the end of his letter, Michael wrote: "You will get through this." I treasured his words and carried the letter in my purse for several months as a good luck charm.

With Broffman's letter came a long recipe for herbs, written in Chinese. This was accompanied by instructions in English on how to prepare and take them. I was to pass the recipe on to Bob Flaws, who would make up the herb blends.

First, though, we sat in his office and talked. Bob Flaws was a slender man, with light brown hair and pale skin stretched like parchment over finely chiseled bones. His eyes were bright blue and transparent: I imagined that he must subsist wholly on fruit, grains, vegetables, purified water and air. He issued his opinions and diagnoses sitting bolt upright in a hard wooden chair in the small, comfortable office he maintained in his home. Everything about him, from his words to his posture, was clear-edged and definite. I knew from Bill that Bob would take on only patients whom he thought he could help, and that he had been known to drop clients who were not responding to treatment or who failed to follow the dietary and lifestyle guidelines he laid out. It was simply against his principles to waste his patients' money or his own time and, like Jim Cleaver and Christa, he deliberately kept his charges low.

I had always been impressed with Bob. I loved the precision of his thinking and his obvious skill. To watch him insert his acupuncture needles was to watch an artist at work. Still, when his wife, Honora Wolfe (herself a healer), told me that Bob's favorite television program was "Miami Vice," I was delighted. It was so reassuring to know that he, too, had his frailties.

The Chinese system is based on a completely different understanding of illness, health and humankind's place in the universe than the one informing our Western system. Like healers from almost all traditional cultures, Chinese doctors believe human beings are part of an entire system: you cannot be altogether well in a sick society or in a sick world. The Chinese see a kind of energy—called *qi* or *chi*—permeating the universe, underlying all phenomena. This same energy courses through our bodies along pathways called meridians. If the flow of energy becomes blocked or distorted, illness results. The purpose of acupuncture, herbs and massage is to free or redirect *qi*.

There is also the polarity between yin and yang; yang is generally defined as expansive, masculine, big, bright, fiery, and yin as feminine, small, dark, interior. Like all things, the organs of the body (which, in Chinese medicine, bear only a very rough correspondence to the organs we Westerners know about) are seen as yin or yang, and so are all foods and herbs. Yin and yang must be brought into balance.

Finally, this system classifies all things as belonging to five elements: wood, fire, earth, metal and water. These elements are not fixed but are constantly evolving, one into another. Nothing, in fact, is static in the Chinese doctor's world, and a good practitioner will continually change and readjust treatments to respond to this dynamic reality.

These theories are not based on empirical evidence: Chinese custom once forbade autopsies and even surgery. The entire schematic was constructed from the observation of physical processes over thousands of years.

A traditional Chinese doctor arrives at a diagnosis by close observation of the patient: skin color, breath, carriage, smell and general appearance. The doctor will also spend a great deal of time listening to the patient's pulse and will ask to examine his or her tongue. As I discovered, Chinese doctors inquire about one's excretory habits in embarrassing detail. These doctors do not see themselves as treating discrete symptoms, but as adjusting the patient's entire system.

Although some experts are now attempting to investigate acupuncture points to determine if they have some unique electro-physical characteristics, Chinese theory remains unverifiable. Nobody has ever seen a meridian. No one has ever documented the process of energy flow. Still, a patient who has ever had an acupuncture needle inserted by a knowledgeable Chinese doctor has felt the body's response, whether as a profound reverberation, a cramping or a kind of electrical tingle. And while the correspondence between acupuncture (or acupressure) spots and the functioning of inner organs may be unprovable, there was a certain place on my shin that, when rubbed by Christa, never failed to make my stomach growl!

Bob told me that the development of cancer is often preceded by a liver ailment. This held true for me, I told him. I had had hepatitis in 1971. He said that that might have been part of the cause, along with an abortion I'd had at twenty-one and my seven years on the birth control pill.

"If a cancer occurs in a relatively external location like the breast or uterus," Bob said, "and you just have it cut out— without addressing the imbalance that caused it in the first place—it will recur deeper in the body."

In a way, this pleased me. It seemed to validate my decision to make do with a lumpectomy. Clearly, radical surgery would not be the Chinese way.

I pulled Michael Broffman's letter from my purse, and Bob read his prescription. "These herbs will do several things for you," he said. "They'll protect your body from some of the bad effects of chemotherapy; they'll shield the integrity of your bone marrow. They will also help expel the poisons from your system."

"Will they work against the chemotherapy? Will they prevent it from doing its job?"

"No. They're designed to be complementary."

I was to take Michael's herbs religiously, said Bob, meditate daily and keep my *qi* moving. "If you're angry," he went on, "don't repress it. But don't lash out, either. Try taking a walk if you can. Here ..." he rummaged in his drawer, "take this tape. Listen to it every day. It'll help you keep your *qi* circulating."

I was also to amend my diet by keeping down my intake of fat (something Western and Chinese doctors agreed on), steering clear of spicy foods, eschewing cheese, coffee and chocolate.

"All chocolate?" I said. "Couldn't I just cut down? I mean, couldn't I just have a piece of chocolate once a week or something?"

Bob's profile was chiseled in stone. "If it were my life that were at stake," he remarked austerely, "I don't think I'd be bargaining over chocolate."

Then he softened a little. "Just relax, take the herbs, follow the diet and listen to this relaxation tape every single day. I'll do the worrying about your illness."

A few days later, I went to Bob's house to pick up the herbs. The size of the box, which had been left on the porch for me, was astonishing. When I got it home, I saw that it contained ten packets, each crammed with what looked like a mixture of bark, twigs, fungi and berries. These herbs, along with the water to simmer them in, barely fit in the largest cooking utensil I could conjure up.

In his letter, Broffman had stipulated that the herbs were to be soaked for forty minutes, simmered for another forty and "boiled gently" for forty more. I never could figure out the difference between simmered and "boiled gently." The cooking process smelled up the house and produced a black liquid, covered with debris. Then the herb water had to be cooled and strained. The entire operation took well over two hours and had to be repeated daily, which meant that I either got up at 5 A.M. to boil herbs or went to work late. I was to drink five cups of the herb water over the course of the day. I'd toss down one cup in the morning and two in the evening. I carried two more cups in separate glass jars to work. "Hey," Ronda Haskins was sure to remark as I came in, "it's the pond scum lady." This process went on for ten days; then I'd get a few days' break and begin again.

It was sometimes pretty difficult. The mixture tasted as revolting as it looked. The reaction it created, going down, was less an impulse to throw up than a kind of inward shuddering, as if all my intestines were in cold recoil. I managed reasonably well on the weeks I was off chemotherapy. But the rest of the time, I'd pour a full glass of the ugly, black liquid and stand by the sink almost in tears, my system heaving from the chemicals, sure I'd vomit up any drop of herb water I managed to choke down.

Fortunately, Bill's stint in the military had prepared him for just this kind of crisis, and he was always available to help. He had his own method. He'd thrust his face out until his nose was inches from mine, the veins in his forehead would pop, his skin would redden. And then he'd explode: "What the fuck's the matter with you, you whimpering piece of shit? You some kind of fucking pussy? You some kind of wimp? Arrrrrright, slimebag, I want those herbs down, and I want 'em down right now. Now, move, dammit. Move. Move. Move. Move. Move. Get that shit down your throat. ..."

I'd end up laughing too hard to swallow.

Bob Flaws had pointed out in his consultation with me that Chinese medicine requires a far more active patient than does Western medicine: If you decide to follow its precepts, you can't just pop a pill or submit to an injection. You have to feel a real belief in the process and a commitment to changing the way you live your life. I was beginning to understand what he meant.

Because he was inexperienced in dealing with cancer patients at that time, Bob Flaws was taking direction from Michael Broffman and following the herb protocols Broffman prescribed to the letter. The communication between them didn't seem to be ideal, however. Michael was telling me on the phone that the herb formulas had to be changed regularly and that Bob should see me weekly and modify the brew as needed. Bob didn't seem to feel this was necessary. In the meantime, operating on the general principle that a second opinion was always useful—as it had proved when I was deciding on surgery and chemotherapy—I paid a visit to Christa's doctor, a young Chinese woman whose patients called her Dr. Lin.

She seemed a little puzzled by the visit, and, because of her broken English, we had some difficulty in communicating. But I showed her Michael's prescription, she seemed to approve it, and I left. A week or so later she called, very emphatic and insistent. Was someone changing the herb prescription? she wanted to know. Herbs had to be changed periodically, in response to changes in the body. "Is not good to keep same all the time. Must change," she said emphatically.

"What am I supposed to do?" I asked Michael on the phone. "Bob doesn't seem to want to see me regularly, you're trying to treat me long distance and Dr. Lin is insistent that the herbs be modified."

"If she's willing to change the prescription," Michael said, "go to her."

The problem was that now Dr. Lin didn't want to take me. She was extremely busy, having acquired a kind of mild cult status in Boulder. More important, she felt I was Michael's and Bob's patient, and that to take me on was to demonstrate a lack of respect for her colleagues.

"You don't understand," I kept explaining, "they want you to help me. They recommended I see you."

Finally, she relented.

Dr. Lin had been trained in Western medicine in China, selected by the government to become a doctor during the Cultural Revolution. Six years later she was picked out again: Traditional Chinese practice had been all but obliterated during the Cultural Revolution, and now the government wanted it revived. She studied the ancient theory, then apprenticed to practitioners, learning herbology, acupuncture and *tuina*, Chinese massage.

"It's really important to follow a special doctor and learn in his way, and he can tell you his personal experience," she told me at one point. "In Western medicine, you diagnose from symptoms, exams and laboratory work. In Chinese medicine, the diagnosis could vary according to the different teachers."

She studied herbs with one doctor who was seventy-five years old and had a lifetime of observation to impart. "There are thousands of different herbs," she said. "You not only need to remember the names, you need be very familiar with the characteristics. Each herb is different on its own, and when several herbs are combined, they can increase the result. Some herbs will contradict others. And some have side effects. So you need to be careful."

The acupuncturist who taught her came from a long line of practitioners. "They have family secrets. I am very lucky he taught me. I feel very honored."

Lin had found that practicing medicine in the United States required some adjustment. "The American body, the structure is the same, but the emotions and life habits, the food—all different—and also the rhythms."

I learned there were Boulder physicians who sent patients to Dr. Lin. There was even one young doctor whom she had helped become pregnant.

The herb regime she recommended for me was a little easier than Michael Broffman's. The packages were smaller, and I was permitted to soak the herbs overnight and simmer them for only forty minutes in the morning, which was a big improvement. She did stipulate that I was not to use an aluminum pot.

The lifestyle changes she prescribed, however, were more far-reaching than anything that had been suggested before. She echoed Bob's prohibition on coffee, cheese, chocolate, spicy foods. She forbade me to drink alcohol. (The only time I ever saw her angry was a year and a half after this first visit, when I told her I'd had three or four piña coladas on a week-long vacation in Hawaii. I knew she was angry, though she didn't stop smiling. As a warning, she told me a terrible story about a woman who'd had a recurrence of breast cancer and died.) She also wanted me to avoid beef and veal, lamb and mutton, and all kinds of fish except those, like catfish, salmon and trout, that swam in rivers. I could eat shellfish—clams, mussels and oysters—but not lobster, crab or shrimp. Above all, I was not to touch chicken or eggs, though I could eat turkey, duck or any other fowl. Periodically, half in fun, half in earnest, I'd test my boundaries. "Can I eat elk, Dr. Lin?" "Yes." "Buffalo?" "Sure."

"Why no chicken?"

"In China, cancer people not eat chicken. Chicken not good for cancer people."

Eventually, she told me that that particular prohibition was not based on any principles of yin or yang, balance or heat and cold. It was scientific.

"We did tests in China. In laboratories. We find out that if cancer cells present, chicken or eggs make them grow."

"But if that's the case, why don't Western doctors know about it?"

"They don't believe us. They don't believe our statistics."

Michael Broffman pointed out some time later that chickens are highly susceptible to tumors. "Of course," he said, "we don't know which diseases can translate from chickens to people. But chickens can catch colds from us. So who knows?"

A waitress once told me that it was irritating to work in Boulder because the town was so full of self-absorbed health and fitness fanatics. They'd ask for water without ice, salads without dressing, pecan nuts instead of blueberries in their pancakes— myriad special requests that required extra work on her part. Now, somewhat shamefacedly, I joined these people's ranks.

"Is this asparagus soup vegetarian?" I'd ask a harried waiter. "Or does it have a chicken broth base? Is there mayonnaise in your salad dressing? Does this iced tea have caffeine in it?" In particular, it was difficult to avoid eggs, which seemed to pop up in everything I loved, from muffins to gourmet noodles. In restaurants, I'd scan the menus for entrees containing none of the forbidden meats—and find that the one vegetarian offering was smothered in cheese.

In the first weeks after my cancer diagnosis, I was highly suggestible—almost in a state of trance. So food seemed to offer magical possibilities of salvation, as well as untold dangers. I became preoccupied with what I ate and with what I prepared for my family. I created vegetarian dishes—ratatouilles, potato curries, spaghetti sauces piquant with basil and rich with exotic mushrooms.

But then I read about macrobiotic diets, which ban eggplant, tomatoes and potatoes. "Basil," said a medical student friend, "contains a high level of natural carcinogens." A local scientist said the same about mushrooms (previously, I had read that exotic mushrooms had antitumor activity) and all sprouts. All the self-help books seemed to agree that salmon helped prevent cancer, but a cancer patient I met said he'd seen a study in which mice who already had tumors worsened when fed the omega-3 fatty acids present in the fish.

"All right," I said finally, slamming down the cookbook I'd been skimming. "I'll just stop eating altogether."

Eventually, I forged a diet high in fruits and vegetables, low in fat, and containing foods generally considered to have some anticancer activity: green and licorice root tea; foods high in beta-carotenes, like sweet potatoes, cantaloupe and carrots; garlic; cruciferous vegetables like broccoli and cabbage; rye breads and crackers; strawberries; kiwi fruit. And sometimes I cheated.

Bill and Anna declared flatly that they had no intention of following my ridiculous diet. But that didn't prevent me from constantly urging them to avoid hamburgers and teasing them mercilessly about the white slime on their tongues.

There were other aspects of Chinese practice that aroused cynicism in the West. Lin was horrified, for example, when she found out that no one had asked me about my menstrual cycle before performing surgery. She said that it was very bad to operate on someone who was menstruating. I have since seen Western studies that bear her out; at least one, from Italy, indicated that undergoing breast cancer surgery while menstruating made recurrence more likely, and a second study showed that it was best to have surgery while ovulating.

Dr. Lin also suggested it would be better if chemotherapy did not take place on days when I had my period—an injunction that was sometimes difficult to follow and that John Fleagle found plain ridiculous.

I had read in Western magazines that researchers were trying to discover if there was an optimal time of day for receiving chemotherapy. Is there a particular hour when cancer cells are most apt to be dividing and hence most susceptible to being destroyed? Lin suffered no ambivalence on the topic. "You have treatments at ten in morning," she told me.

Lin could not have been more unlike the ascetic Bob Flaws. She was a little dumpling of a woman, quick to smile and laugh and fond of teasing. "You like these herbs better," she'd say, making out the prescription in tiny Chinese characters. "I put in some chocolate."

An engineering student (she hoped eventually to help establish the physical basis of acupuncture), Lin lived with her husband and her mother in one of the small, student apartments near the university. The place was colorful and cluttered: carpet, curtains, armchairs and sofa were covered in autumnal patterns of brown and orange, but all the patterns were different, and the colors varied slightly from piece to piece. There were ribbons on the lampshades; a low table contained candy dishes and English-language Chinese magazines with bright red covers.

Dr. Lin's eighty-one-year-old mother, dressed in padded black clothes, always sat in front of the television set, a shawl over her shoulders. She fiddled periodically with an array of small objects on a tray in front of her—a saucer of snacks, green and gold boxes of pills. Whenever I turned in her direction, she smiled and nodded.

On every visit, I sat by Dr. Lin at the kitchen table. On the wall across from me was a sand painting with figures representing health and fertility—a gift from a patient. There was also a peaceful black-and-white photograph of swans. A small glass on the table contained acupuncture needles in an alcohol solution. A stuffed green Kermit the Frog, wrapped in a paper towel, served as a resting place for my wrist while Dr. Lin took my pulse—first on the right hand, then on the left.

Now, an Oriental doctor taking a pulse is a wondrous thing. In his beautiful book of essays, *Mortal Lessons: Notes on the Art of Surgery*, Richard Selzer speaks of watching the Dalai Lama's doctor, Yeshi Dhonden, taking a pulse. "From the foot of the bed, where I stand, it is as though he and the patient have entered a special place of isolation, of apartness, about which a vacancy hovers, and across which no violation is possible." Then he observes, "I know that I, who have palpated a hundred thousand pulses, have not felt a single one."

Yeshi Dhonden, incidentally, made his diagnosis solely from the pulse-taking and from inhaling the odor of the patient's urine. This is how he phrased his diagnosis, according to Selzer: "Between the chambers of her heart, long, long before she was born, a wind had come and blown open a deep gate that must never be opened. Through it charge the full waters of her river, as the mountain stream cascades in the springtime. ..." His diagnosis was correct.

The way the Western doctors put it? "Congenital heart disease ... interventricular septal defect, with resultant heart failure."

Now I would not have described Dr. Lin as poised above my wrist "like some exotic golden bird with folded wings." But she did become gravely concentrated for many minutes at a time, tapping with small, dry fingers on my wrist, now lightly, now with more pressure. I knew that she felt for three pulses on each wrist and found a rhythm beneath each finger, and at every level of pressure. It was as if, where Western doctors heard only the piping of a tin whistle, she were monitoring the sounds of an orchestra.

I asked her once what she was feeling for, and, like other Chinese doctors, she seemed to find words inadequate to describe it. "I can check rate, strength, quality," she said, "and also—it's hard to explain—a deepness or exploding. ..."

Lin's kindness and affection seemed part of her practice. She always hugged me before I left, murmuring, "Be well, Julia." Once she added, "I love you."

I called her one Wednesday evening. I had a fairly violent stomach flu: my guts were knotted, I was nauseated. She told me to come over the next day and, when I arrived, handed me two green and gold boxes containing vials of pellets. She wanted no money for them. She hadn't had time to order any herbs, so she was giving me some medication relatives had sent from China for her mother's sometimes queasy stomach. Because of the political situation there, she didn't know when she could get any more.

"I can't take these," I protested.

"It is necessary for you to be well," she said, pressing the vials into my hand. "I want you should be very well."

I will never know how much Lin's herbs were responsible for the fact that I came through the chemotherapy strongly and well. But for minor ailments, her remedies were clearly very effective. The pills she gave me eased my stomach within hours. She could also adjust my herb prescription so that, for example, I would urinate more or less frequently. If I complained to her that my sleep was restive, broken by nightmares, she'd concoct a potion that sent me into a deep and dreamless slumber.

127

There were awed Boulderites who found her ministrations mystical or exotic, yet Lin herself was unfailingly practical and down-to-earth. Once I came early for a session. As I relaxed on her couch with a highly colored Chinese magazine, scanning an article about a shoe factory, she took the pulse of a slender young man.

"Wow," he said. "You know, I think I can finally feel what it is that's happening in my body, what you're listening for. All the pulses and rhythms. It's like they're answering your fingers."

I was impressed. "I've never felt that," I told Dr. Lin when my turn came around. "I've never felt anything at all when you took my pulse."

She had an odd look on her face, as if she were pursing her lips so as not to laugh. Finally, she said diplomatically, "He must be very sensitive young man. I never feel these things with my doctor either."

11
AMAZONS AND ANGELS

I was sitting in John Day's office after a routine checkup while he congratulated me on my progress.

"You look so much better," he said. "Lighter. Both physically and mentally."

I was pleased. "It's this insane diet. Almost no fat. And there's so little I'm allowed to eat ..."

"Well, whatever it is, it's clearly doing you good. And I'm glad you're doing everything you can, working with Chinese medicine and everything. You know, you had that freaky, aggressive kind of tumor ..."

"What?"

"We told you that."

"No, you didn't. Nobody did."

"Now, Juliet," he said, "you're getting all stressed out again. You're going to be all right."

"But nobody said anything about an aggressive tumor." I felt as if a huge block of concrete were pressing against my chest.

"Well," said Dr. Day, "let's see." He began thumbing through my chart. As he did, Candis called through the door that he was wanted in surgery.

"I've got to go," he said. "I can't find it now. You'll be OK, I tell you."

Back at work, I stared unseeing at my computer screen. Finally, I called and left a message for John Fleagle. "What kind of tumor did I have?" I asked when he called back. "Why did Dr. Day say it was a peculiarly aggressive one? What was he talking about?"

"What you had," he responded, "was common, or garden variety, breast cancer. Nothing more or less, nothing exceptionally

129

aggressive. The statistics I quoted to you the first time we talked still apply. Now relax and enjoy the weekend."

In a passing spasm of paranoia, I wondered if the doctors shared some information on my illness so terrible that they were conspiring to keep it from me. But then I decided that John Day must simply have confused my case briefly with that of another patient. I pushed the incident to the back of my mind. It was several months before I found out what he'd been talking about.

It did seem odd, though, that I had found the words "common or garden variety cancer" so reassuring. A few months earlier, a diagnosis of any kind of cancer had seemed the ultimate horror. Now it was turning out there were gradations of horror. "Yup," said a friend to whom I described this incident, "and the garden variety can kill you just as effectively as any other kind."

In the weeks following my diagnosis I had discovered that Jean Paul Sartre was right: Hell is other people. Heaven is other people, too. Once you know you have cancer, you enter a different world. You feel like an alien, or someone who's just been dropped onto the indifferent face of the moon. As you carry your illness out into the world, people look to you for cues. How do you want to be spoken to? You often feel like the host at a difficult party. You make little jokes to lighten the atmosphere.

I recognized the dynamics clearly some time later, when a friend was diagnosed as having breast cancer. She was describing a conversation with her lover just before Halloween. It was about the fact that she'd decided to eat huge quantities of vegetables in the hope of shoring up her health.

"He said I'd soon be turning green," she said. "And I told him, 'Well, Juliet's turning orange from all the carrots she's eating. We can go to costume parties together as a salad.'"

Later she said that she and her lover would be able to deal with her mastectomy just fine: "After all, we have another whole breast to play with."

I loved her gallantry, her grace under pressure, but I recognized its source from my own early months. Being brave and keeping your sense of humor, having everyone say, "Isn't Juliet strong?

Isn't she being wonderful?" and seeing their relief because you've eased their interaction with you—all that is a way of dealing with the fear. I recognized the shakiness, the kind of feverish cast to my friend's humor. I knew that the little jokes she floated during the day didn't prevent the wakeful gray mornings when she sobbed aloud in fear, begged God to let her live.

There were people who didn't need a cue from me, who stepped naturally and easily into the role of comforter. A novelist friend left a tape of soothing piano music on my desk at work with a note: "When things go bad for me, I listen to Michael Jones. He changes one's brainwaves. I really believe this." The day before my surgery he dropped off a card: "I've been thinking of you— which is the closest I get to prayer—and hoping for the best." A co-worker whom I barely knew bought me a copy of Jill Ireland's *Life Wish*. With it she put a bright pink notepad. Each page contained a drawing of a naked man with no genitalia. This pad was for doodling. I treasured all the cards and letters I received, packing them away carefully in a drawer.

I remembered the morning early on when a black friend, Virginia Williams, came to the house. She took one look at my face and asked what was troubling me. "I have breast cancer," I said and broke into tears. I was in her arms in an instant. "Come to my church," she murmured. "Come to church with me. They will heal you there."

I was overwhelmed at the ubiquity and immensity of simple human kindness. And I was astonished by the warmth and generosity of a number of women, some of whom were old friends, some new acquaintances. In the late sixties and early seventies, I had spoken glibly about universal sisterhood—a kind of mystic bond between all women. Now I found this concept was true in ways I could never have imagined before. There were the mind-steadying weekly calls from Doris Olsen; there was Diana Somerville's instant help and understanding the day I heard about the bad mammogram; there was the friend who saw that I was crying in the middle of a movie and simply took my hand and kept it in a strong, warm grip for the rest of the evening; there was Kathryn Bernheimer, grilling her doctor cousin about the best treatments, the best local doctors. Later, in Aspen, there would be Caryn McVoy, whose sorrowful memories of her own father's death from cancer did not prevent her from driving me to chemotherapy sessions two Wednesdays in a row and holding my hand as the drugs were administered.

And there was Jeannie Fuller. The wife of a prominent Colorado Republican, she had served on the board of the Colorado Council on the Arts and Humanities when I was a staff member there. She was a thoughtful, competent, pretty woman, who flew her own small plane. I remembered hearing that she had breast cancer, and shortly after that she left the board, and I lost track of her. As far as I knew, she was still alive, so I added her to the little list of names I kept playing and replaying in my mind of women who had survived breast cancer.

Now she called out of the blue. She had heard about my plight from a mutual acquaintance.

"Oh, Jeannie," I said, surprised at my own enthusiasm, "I've been thinking about you."

"Of course you have," she said.

"Well, you know," I blurted, "because you're still alive and ..." I stopped. Had I just been unpardonably rude?

But Jeannie laughed. "I am alive," she said. "And it's been six years. I feel terrific. And you're going to be fine, too."

She began telling me what to expect as the chemotherapy progressed. She had been on the same protocol for a year. "My doctor told me back then that it appeared that six months' worth of treatment would be as effective as a year's worth. But they weren't completely sure. The figures weren't all in. And, of course, I wanted to be safe."

She told me that she'd jogged regularly that year; that she'd been able to cope well with the nausea; that her hair had thinned but not fallen out: "So I was able to get away with a very short cut, but no wig." She warned me about the depression patients seem to experience somewhere in the middle of the protocol. "And you'll find you have vaginal dryness," she told me briskly, going on to recommend ointments.

I was surprised and delighted by her candor—"I was discussing vaginal dryness with a Republican today," I told Bill at dinner that evening—but I was finding that it was not unusual. The information I received from fellow patients was invariably more detailed, rich and specific than anything my doctors ever told me, and these women could supply a special kind of comfort, too.

Doris Olsen once told me that she'd been fretting about what a mastectomy actually looked like some time before her surgery. She mentioned this to a visiting friend who had also had breast cancer. The friend pulled the blind down over the window. "It looks like this," she said, and opened her blouse.

I received some distinctly unhelpful responses, too. One came from a local artist: "Well, it can't be very bad," she said, interrupting my description of the treatments I was undergoing. "Not if they're letting you keep your breast." A gay friend sighed when I told him my news. "I'm going to a funeral Sunday," he said. "Seems like it's nothing but funerals these days."

"I'm not exactly dead," I snapped.

There were many New Age people who called to say something like, "If you really want to be well, you will"—a comment that inspired in me a near-irresistible desire to slam down the phone. A few friends completely stopped calling. One or two periodically asked mutual acquaintances about my health, with an apologetic: "I know I should call her, but I don't know what to say." One of these people explained many months later that he had known a woman who'd died of breast cancer. He was afraid that if he spoke to me, he'd somehow let that fact slip out.

"Were you under the impression that I'd never considered the possibility of dying?" I asked him. "Or that the fear of death hasn't been with me every second, day and night, since the moment I heard my diagnosis? Nothing you could have said or let slip could have hurt me as much as your silence."

To be sure, talking to a newly diagnosed cancer patient can be a ticklish business. I knew that. It isn't as if we are all the same. And obviously we need different kinds of help at different stages in our treatment and thinking. Many patients I met confirmed

133

this. During the "brave and wonderful" stage, pulsating expressions of sympathy undermined the control we were desperately fighting to achieve. But that didn't mean we wanted our very real fears and sorrows unacknowledged. In other words, I concluded, it was fine to say, "I'm so sorry about what's happening to you"— but not in the tearful, quavering tones suitable for a eulogy.

I loved stories about a sister, friend, mother, aunt who had survived breast cancer and lived into old age, but not when the details were unconvincing. And while at times I shied away from any thoughts of death and dying, at other times I wanted to discuss the possibility and resented people who said too rapidly, "Oh, you're not going to die." If it was said with real affection, however, the statement was reassuring. Sometimes I called up Caryn McVoy in Carbondale just to hear her say, "I know you're going to be fine. I'm not worried about you."

Any gesture that bespoke real caring—from a gift certificate to the local ice cream shop to a funny card—called forth deep gratitude. Any friend who made a point of being available at this time—no matter what he or she did or said—was a friend for life.

The almost universal comment from those who see a cancer patient on her feet and active is, "Oh, you look wonderful!" This is warm and encouraging, but there's a subtext we recognize: "And here I was expecting you to be emaciated, bald, in agony and gasping for breath." Despite this, I was always heartened by these compliments. I knew other cancer patients, however, who responded with bitter, if unexpressed, derision.

Many of my friends and acquaintances, spurred by what had happened to me, made appointments with their own doctors for mammograms. I was, of course, glad of this, and glad when none of those mammograms showed anything suspicious. Still, I didn't need the flood of details that many of these women insisted on providing.

An acquaintance called to share her relief with me. "I was so scared waiting for the results," she said. "I just couldn't function the last two days. Couldn't work. Couldn't do anything. And then an hour ago I got a call from the nurse. The minute I heard her voice I just freaked. But she said, 'I'm calling to let you know everything's OK, so you don't have to worry any longer than necessary.' Wasn't that sweet of her? Just to call and let me know? So I'm fine. But for a couple of days there I was a basket case. You can't imagine ..."

Yeah, I said to myself. I think I can.

To be truthful, my reaction to this flood of information on the robust health of my friends' breasts was not unambivalent. Of course, I didn't want anyone else I knew to have breast cancer. I had this silly little joke I was using at the time. "Don't worry," I told one friend before she went in for her mammogram. "You know, only one in ten women gets breast cancer. Well, now I've got mine, I get to pick nine women who'll never get it. So you're completely safe."

But it was also an awful thing to be alone in this universe of relieved and rejoicing women. To be the dreaded example of the one thing they all feared most.

A year later, all these confused and floating feelings coalesced when an old friend found a lump in her breast. I had lunch with her while she awaited the results of her mammogram, and I easily recognized the state she was in, the odd mixture of shaky almost-elation and terror. You're so frantically alive at these times and so yearning for the comfort of your customary half sleep. When the mammogram turned up nothing, she became her old self on the instant, laughing, joyful, confident, not allowing a whisper of what she'd understood about her own mortality to remain in her mind.

I wanted to say to her, "That place you were just in, that place you visited for a few days, that's where I've been living all year, Margaret. That's become my home."

I wanted her to say to me, "Yes, I know. I understand. I finally understand how this has been for you."

That conversation never took place, and, watching her pick up the threads of her daily life again, I was filled with loneliness.

Dr. Fleagle and Patti Kealiher had told me that the chemotherapy might cause my hair to fall out, and I hadn't thought that would bother me very much. I didn't consider myself particularly vain. At one point, I drifted into a rather charming antique clothing store and bought a crimson scarf and a white straw boater. These were intended as jaunty choices, but my mood, paying for them, was grim. And then one night I put my hand to the back of my head and, when I drew it back, found the palm crisscrossed with hairs. I panicked. I saw again the skull-like head of my mother in her last few weeks of life. I saw the emaciated survivors of the Nazi death camps. "Please," I sobbed in Bill's arms, "please don't let me die."

I'd been told that it was best to buy a wig before becoming bald: once you were, it was hard, other cancer patients said, even to leave the house to shop for one. Then, if it turned out you didn't need the wig after all (most patients on the protocol I was enduring found that their hair thinned but did not fall out entirely), the worst that would happen is that you'd possess a new fashion accessory. The next morning I called a Denver wig-fitter Patti Kealiher had recommended and made an appointment for a fitting. "My name is Mary Franks," said the oddly prim and formal voice on the phone. "Just come in, and I'll be waiting for you." I called my friend Diana Somerville, and she offered to drive me there.

At around ten the next morning, we arrived at a half-deserted shopping center on the outskirts of Denver. The wig-fitters, identified by a hand-lettered cardboard sign that said "Linda's Boutique," seemed to be one of only a handful of functioning businesses in the complex.

Linda's Boutique was a small, cluttered store, crammed with odd knickknacks and articles of clothing. There were cut-glass vases, cheap figurines, a china goose wearing a blue china jacket. In one window, an improbably golden wig gleamed on a stand. Diana and I glanced rapidly at each other, contemplating a hasty retreat, but Mary Franks had seen us and was coming forward to help.

She was dark and slender, her hair and dress preternaturally tidy. Behind her I saw another woman, with fluffed-out, bright blonde hair. The entire milieu looked like the cluttered set for one of Tennessee Williams's charged and eccentric one-act plays.

But then Mary Franks was settling me into a chair and running her fingers thoughtfully through my thinning hair. And immediately—as under John Day's hands or John Fleagle's—I found myself relaxing. Her touch alone made her expertise clear.

On the seat next to mine, an elderly woman was being fitted with a dark brown wig. It looked obviously artificial. "I think," Mary Franks's co-worker was murmuring, "that perhaps you need something a little lighter, a little closer to your own hair color."

The old woman was clearly enamored of the wig. "How about you," she said in our general direction, "what do you think?"

As tactfully as possible, Diana and I seconded Mary Franks's partner. And for the next fifteen minutes, with angelic patience, the partner fitted wigs that shaded from dark brown to pure gray, turned her customer's seat, stood back, held up a mirror, commented. When the woman left, she seemed entirely satisfied with her purchase: a wig a little darker than her own gray hair and a good bit lighter than the one she had originally picked out.

Meanwhile, Mary Franks had studied my hair thoughtfully for a few minutes, then vanished into the back room. She returned with a couple of wigs that were short, professional-looking, rather like my own cut.

"We actually need to go a shade or two lighter than your real hair," she explained. "The hair on a wig is so dense, that if you get it in the exact same color as your hair, the overall effect is a good bit darker."

The wigs seemed usable, but a bit dull. I asked if I could change my hair color. I'd always wondered how it felt to be blonde or to have red hair. That wasn't advisable, said Franks. A color other than your own almost always looks unnatural: "We'll find something you like."

She made it clear that she was in no hurry, that she had many wigs in different sizes and colors in the back room, that she was also prepared to special order should nothing on hand suit me.

"I don't want this to look artificial," I said. I'd had nightmares of looking freaky, of people whispering as they passed me in the street: "Poor woman. You know she has cancer." I didn't want pity. I didn't want to be excluded from the human race. "I don't mind how much I have to pay to get one that looks natural."

"We can do that for you at eighty or ninety dollars," said Mary Franks. "You don't have to pay an arm and a leg. The only reason to spend a couple of hundred dollars is if you're buying a wig that has to last, something you intend to wear for years. Also," she added, "you should check and see if your insurance pays for this. Some companies do."

"This one's just kind of to check the color," she added, popping a wig on my head.

I looked in the mirror. There was my face, framed in a wild and wicked tangle of brown curls. I held up my hand as Mary Franks moved to take the wig off.

"Wait a minute," I said. "Oh ... I guess it's ridiculous. But ... hey, Diana, what do you think?"

"I like it."

The person in the mirror wasn't the strained sad woman who had lain awake all night thinking about death. She was cheerful and frivolous, bouncy and curly. The sheer volume of her hair was astonishing.

"Could I get away with this?"

Mary Franks was smiling. "Let me work with it a little. You girls can just get a cup of tea somewhere and come back in an hour. Then you'll see."

There was a friendly health food store next door to Linda's Boutique, and Diana and I whiled away the time in a quiet corner, with steaming cups of peppermint tea. Then we returned.

The wig had been shaped and trimmed back a little, and Franks placed it on my head and began working again. She tousled, arranged, snipped, and as she did she passed on vital information, things that in my fear and confusion I hadn't even thought to ask about.

She suggested I buy a couple of light, colorful caps for jogging or swimming. She said that the wig was pretty well fitted, but it could fly off if, say, I were walking across a windy parking lot with an armload of groceries. "Try to keep one hand free to hold it down," she said. She instructed me in how to wash the wig, how to create a stand for it (two soda cans taped together), how to comb it out: "It's not like real hair. The curls just tend to spring back." She told me that if I wanted any changes in the look after wearing the wig a few days or weeks, I could return to her and she'd restyle it.

Then she started talking about her work. She had spent twenty years working with cancer patients, and in that time she'd learned a lot. She told me about women who'd had mastectomies and then been deserted by their husbands.

"That's terrible," said Diana. "Imagine having to deal with your marriage breaking up when you're still reeling from finding out you have cancer. I mean, I guess a woman is best rid of a guy like that, but still ..."

"The timing of it ... ," I said.

"That's right," said Mary Franks. "But it does happen."

Though I'd known it before, I suddenly realized full force how lucky I was to have Bill and Anna. I thought about women who had no partner or an unsympathetic one, no co-workers, no close-knit circle of friends. Old women alone in dusty rooms. Young women alone with little children. Women without insurance, waiting for care in crowded emergency rooms. How did they get through something like this?

Franks said she was seeing more and more breast cancer patients, and they were coming to her younger and younger: "It used to be," she said, "that I never saw anyone under sixty. Then it was under fifty. Now I'm used to seeing women in their forties. In the last six weeks, I've seen twenty-five women who were under thirty-five. The youngest was twenty-four." I thought about the birth control pill and shuddered.

"There," said Mary Franks, her hands hovering about my head. "What do you think?"

I loved it.

"What do we do now?" I asked. "Do you wrap it up or something?"

She drew herself up. "Absolutely not," she said. "You keep this wig on your head, and you go back to your office, and you enjoy it. Get used to it. You don't want to wait until one morning all your hair comes out in the shower or on your brush, and you're standing in front of the mirror crying and hating everything, especially the wig. That starts you out in a whole bad way. Wear it now. Have fun with it. Then when you need it, you'll be prepared." As it turned out, this was excellent advice.

Diana dropped me off at the newspaper. I hesitated a few moments, then walked in to my department. "Hey," said one of the writers, "I love the way you've got your hair done. What is it, a perm? It's really great."

I drew a breath of relief.

Actually, once I'd owned that it was a wig, my hair—and the new identity it gave me—became the topic of fairly intense discussion.

"It's a great look," said one of the reporters. "Sort of divinely sluttish."

"I think it makes me look like an extra on 'The Dolly Parton Show,'" I volunteered. "I ought to have long red fingernails and a fringed jacket and be strumming a guitar."

"I don't agree," said Kathryn Bernheimer. "Not at all. It makes you look like one of those suburban women. Someone with a station wagon full of kids."

I wore the wig for two more weeks. During that time, I bought some new clothes: a bright yellow blouse with a silky, flowered skirt; a very short khaki skirt with a brown and beige, jungle-print shirt. Thanks to Dr. Lin's diet, I was now fairly slender, and I was enjoying this new persona. Finally, I decided that I didn't need the wig. Although I still found alarming quantities of hair in the tub after a shower or on Christa's white mattress when I went for a massage, I seemed to be thinning, rather than going entirely bald. I decided that a short, stylish haircut would suffice for the time being, and I called my regular hairstylist, Robert Dakota.

I did this with some trepidation. Robert was so very elegant. How would he react if he were working on me and quantities of my hair came out in his hands?

"I'm, er, shedding quite a bit," I told him on the phone. "Will that bother you?"

Of course it wouldn't, he said. Come right on in.

Whenever I saw Robert Dakota, Hamlet's line about "a delicate and tender prince" came into my mind. Robert was gentle and soft-spoken but very powerful in his realm. He was much in demand as a stylist, and sometimes it took months to get an appointment with him. Then, as you sat in the waiting area of the smartly decorated, red, gray and black salon, he'd glide over to you—a slender young man in a silky white shirt, black pants, a belt with a curved silver buckle, long ringlets falling to his shoulders. He'd touch your head with soft little dabs, like a kitten tentatively patting a ball of yarn. "Hmmnnn," he'd say, pulling gently at a curl, "it just wants to ... tangle."

When I arrived this time, he greeted me and told me that the wig, which I was wearing for his inspection, was not bad at all. I was relieved to have passed muster. Once I'd taken the wig off, donned a protective smock and had my hair washed, he led me to his chair and began work. I told him something of the saga of the last two months, about some of the help I'd received, and that I was thinking about attending a three-day QuaLife workshop. It turned out that he knew QuaLife director Sara Wolfe—to me, still just a voice on the phone.

"She lost all her hair," he told me. "But she never wore a wig. Just a big silk scarf. She's a beautiful girl. Tall and pretty and blonde. She made a stunning baldie."

It seemed that Sara had lost her job, and her insurance with it, when her boss found out she had cancer. While still on chemotherapy, she decided to run a local race, the Bolder Boulder, and to collect pledges from her friends for doing it. She succeeded beautifully. These same friends also banded together to throw a huge New Year's Eve party as a fundraiser.

"She came in a diaper and T-shirt as the new year," said Robert, "with nothing on her head at all. Bald and shining."

"She must be very brave," I said. "And she must have a wonderful sense of humor."

141

"Yes," he said, "and even dressed like that, she was still gorgeous."

We fell into our customary, comfortable chat: about his brother, who worked on a newspaper in Minnesota, about his newest hobby, which was making videos. I told him how Anna was doing in her dance classes and asked his advice about teachers: his wife, Anne, was also a dancer. Periodically, we fell into a companionable silence, flavored with the scent of the shampoos and unguents he used. He worked without urgency, moving with a dreamlike concentration and precision, like someone administering a sacrament.

I drifted in the chair, looking out of the huge picture window. Since I always had to remove my glasses while Robert worked, the trees, flowers and passers-by on the Boulder Creek pathway seemed at once exceptionally brilliant and comfortingly fuzzy. I received all the daubs at my head, the snippings and combings and touslings, with deep satisfaction, like a cat being caressed behind the ears.

"There," said Robert, turning my chair toward the big mirror, holding a hand mirror behind my head.

Gone was the Dolly Parton extra. My hair was now very very short. A smart, New Yorkish, arty kind of short. It was a haircut that only a very self-confident woman would wear.

"I ... I think I like it," I said. "It's sort of tough-looking. I do. I like it a lot."

"It's your little jock look," said Robert.

As I was paying for the haircut, he walked over to me. In his hand was a beautiful pink stone.

"It's rose quartz." He began wiping it with the corner of a towel. "It'll bring you luck. In money, mostly, but in other things, too. Here, I've wiped my vibrations off it." And he placed it in my palm.

I slipped the smooth, warm stone into my purse.

When I returned to the features department at the newspaper, my co-workers applauded. "It's better than the wig," said David Menconi. "That made it seem like you were trying to look younger than you are."

Driving home, the car window wide open, I marveled at the feel of the wind riffling my hair, the cool, free comfort of my suddenly wigless head.

"The thing that amazes me," I said to Bill at dinner, "is how all these people have appeared in the last three months to help me. Some of them I've known all along, and some I didn't know at all. Robert and Diana and Dr. Wood and the wig lady. Every time I think I'm completely lost, every time I'm really drowning and frightened and desperate, somebody appears and holds out a hand to help me back to shore."

12
STRIKING OUT

One night I had a nightmare. I dreamed there was a fledgling on a high ledge. It was skeletal and blackened, as if it had been burnt, and I knew it was dying. Anna was dying, too. She was as thin and weak as the bird. Still, she was trying to climb up to the ledge to help it. Only every time she came close, she fell back, weak and exhausted.

Then I was sitting in a lecture hall, talking with the people around me about the government violence against the Left during the sixties—a violence that has largely been washed out of our communal memory. The audience was skeptical. A friend with whom I'd lived in a commune during that period joined me and backed my version of events, and his warmth and straight-forwardness carried a conviction that my agitation could not. I knew this man's father had died of cancer.

Anna walked up to us. She was a little stronger but still very pale. Only now she was in another kind of danger. A shadowy person—someone whom I couldn't see, but who I sensed was present—intended to abduct her. I found a dog leash in my hand and started trying to figure out how to attach it to the loop of her pants so that no one could take her away.

I woke up in tears. Bill was heavily, peacefully asleep. I lay with my eyes fixed on the dark ceiling. I finally understood something I had never fully let myself realize before. Dying would mean losing everything. Dying would mean losing Anna.

Thinking it over in the morning, I had some idea where the image of the bird had come from. Once when Anna was a baby, we had visited Pater. A friend from Israel, Klari, was staying at his house, and she was very much taken with Anna, offering her fragments of dark chocolate (which dissolved all over her cheeks), holding and rocking and crooning to her. "I have a daughter, too," she said, handing me a yellowing snapshot. It showed a young, fashionably dressed Klari with a laughing little girl of three or four.

"She's beautiful," I said. "Where is she now?"

Klari answered in German. She said, "They burned her. They took her when she was six." She said it as simply as that.

And I knew her words had somehow floated into my sleeping mind and been connected there with the name some people give to the Jewish children who perished in the death camps: *fogele*, little birds.

When I took the dream and my terror to Dr. Wood, he reminded me of the insidious effects of the chemotherapy I was on. "It affects your brain," he told me. "It makes you weak and tired, and it affects your emotions. Physically." He stressed the last word, giving the *s* the pleasant sibilance of his Chilean accent. "That's why Anna—who represented you—kept falling back in the dream. But eventually she came back, stronger, just as you will when the treatments are over."

I found that useful to hold on to. It meant I wasn't going crazy. From my conversations with other women, I was discovering that depression and extreme anxiety were among chemotherapy's cornucopia of side effects, and few doctors seemed aware of this, or thought to warn their patients about it.

In August, Bill quit his job as planned and decided to enjoy a few weeks of leisure before looking for consulting work. He began learning to relax, even taking up golf so that he could go to Denver occasionally and play with his father. We were visited shortly by some old friends from our graduate student years: Arnie and Alanna Preussner and their daughter Amy, who, at nine, was a year younger than Anna. They joined us in our porch discussions, we all scrapped amiably over newspaper sections in the morning, Alanna applied her considerable culinary skills to creating wonderful dishes that would fit my peculiar diet: a vegetable and tofu stir-fry, a salmon salad with olive oil and crisp pieces of celery and apple. Meanwhile, Amy and Anna were rediscovering their every-summer friendship.

One morning the girls decided to cook us breakfast, with Anna as the chef, Amy as her assistant. Sitting on the porch, we heard a lot of whispering and giggling in the kitchen, and then Anna appeared in the doorway. "Breakfast is served," she said formally. She and Amy began carrying plates out to us: They had peeled and cubed potatoes, sautéing them with mushrooms, tomatoes and garlic. "They're just like you make them," said Anna, "except we put in a handful of slivered almonds. Is it good?" We assured her, quite truthfully, that it was. As we ate, the girls hovered solicitously by us, offering seconds, filling our glasses with orange juice, removing the plates when we were done.

When I came home from work that evening, there was a sign on the front door: "Bed and Brekfast." Amy and Anna, clearly flushed with the success of their cooking that morning, had decided to go into the hospitality business.

"May I show you to your room?" asked Anna, while Amy giggled into a chubby fist. They led me and Bill to our own bedroom, which now had a sign on the door: "Room 402."

After dinner, the girls brought out cookies and cups of tea. Then they escorted all four adults on a triumphant walk down the dirt road at the side of the house, pointing out objects of interest along the way: "And here on our right is Shorty. He's a great horse. Part Arabian, but kinda small. You can feed him some grass if you like. ..."

"If you pull one of these honeysuckle flowers, and take that green thing off the end, you can suck out a bit of honey. ..."

"Don't mind Kaiser. He always barks like that, but he doesn't really mean it."

I had decided to attend the ten-day Aspen Writers' Conference that summer; an author whose first novel I'd very much admired was teaching, and I wanted to study with her. I remembered reading some of her sentences over and over, marveling at their flow and harmony. They came as close to Shakespeare as anything I'd ever seen in prose—if you could classify them as prose at all.

Dr. Fleagle thought getting away would be a good idea and found the timing of the trip perfect: the conference occurred in the middle of my six months of chemotherapy, generally the most difficult period. "It'll take your mind off things," he said. "And I can set it up so a doctor in Aspen administers your chemo for you."

I was excited, but a little nervous. I hadn't been away from Bill and Anna since the diagnosis. Anna would have left for summer camp by the time I got back from Aspen, so that we would not reconnect for a whole month. And I couldn't imagine anyone but Patti Kealiher—who, after all, knew the back of my hand like the back of her hand—administering my chemotherapy drugs.

Patti put together a package for me: tubes of the yellow and white chemotherapy liquids, another tube of saline, the paraphernalia for administration. "I'm sure he'll have some of this stuff," she said when I went to pick it up, "but I just wanted to be safe."

"Will he know exactly what to do?" I asked her. "Did you tell him the sequence, and when the saline goes in and everything?"

Patti laughed. "He's a doctor, Juliet, and giving this chemo isn't a very hard thing to do. It's not exactly brain surgery."

Then I contemplated the problem of Dr. Lin's Chinese herbs. The organizers of the writers' conference had arranged for the students to stay in a group of condominiums, four of us to a unit. One of my roommates would be an old friend, Celeste White, whom I'd met at an earlier conference. But there would also be two strangers. I wasn't sure how these people would feel about waking every morning to the voodoo smell of herbs simmering. Dr. Lin was adamant, however, that I needed to continue taking them.

"You'll just have to tell your roommates why you're doing it," said Bill. "I'm sure they'll understand."

Anna was to stay with Arnie, Alanna and Amy while Bill drove me up to Aspen. The night before I left, she handed me one of her stuffed animals, a brown and white dog with a blunt, mild face.

"Her name's Theresa," Anna said. "I've been sleeping with her for a couple of weeks now, so she's all filled up with Annalove. You can take her to bed with you every night in Aspen."

It was time to leave. Anna trailed me and Bill to the end of the garden path, then hugged me and turned and walked, drooping, back to the house. "I wasn't going to watch you drive away," she said a month later, when the three of us were safely back together. "I thought I'd go crazy if I saw the car leave."

Bill and I drove up to Aspen carrying Patti's care package, my huge, heavy enamel cooking pot, a large box of herbs. Trapped in the car for four hours, I fought depression. In front of my half-seeing eyes, the glorious scenery of route I-70 unreeled: first the sunflowers beaming at the side of the road, the gentle hills, then the piles of rock that looked like building blocks tossed into mounds by a playful giant child. By Lookout Mountain, we saw the outline of hang-gliders against the sky, like hawks. A few miles farther on, a real hawk hung motionless beneath the clouds.

The mountains of Colorado are continually surprising. Through the car windows I'd gaze at a rock face that was clear terra-cotta red, pleated like a lady's fan—and the next outcropping would be gray and drooping, like the patient, wrinkled skin of an elephant. At one point, I watched beige, sandy slopes, dotted with scrub and deciduous trees, slide by to the right of the car, then glanced to the left and saw rolling green hills, reminiscent of the gentler mountains of Europe, peopled by stands of fir trees. In front of us, the slopes were shadowed in melting blues, dark purples and violets, cradling, in places, bright hollows filled with sunlight. All these forms lapped like waves at the foot of the eternal mountain ranges, and, high above us on the granite rocks, shone gleaming lakes of snow.

I should have been profoundly happy. But on clear, fresh days like this one, I'd always find myself wondering whether the nightmare was really receding, or whether I was just enjoying a brief respite, a kind of floating trough between tumultuous waves. Was this the beginning of a normal life, or would the cancer return to engulf me again? As Bill drove, I kept telling myself to focus on the present, on the scenery flowing past the window, on our easy conversation. If this is only a respite, I told myself, why waste it? Why lose precious minutes of living in anticipation of a horror that might or might not come?

Dr. Wood had told me once that in Chile he had heard men joking and laughing in their cells at night, even though they knew they would be tortured in the morning. "And why not?" he had said, with that small, ironic shrug of his. "Should they also have wasted the night?"

Aspen—that rich, beautiful town cradled in the Rocky Mountains—was choked with traffic. Bill became increasingly irritable as we tried, by various routes, to approach the condo I had been assigned. All the roads around it had been torn up and blocked off because of construction on what was to be a huge new hotel. The streets were filled with dust and the sound of jackhammers. Finally, we decided to get lunch and then try approaching the condo again. We parked the car and prepared to walk into town. I glanced back through the window at the plastic bag filled with chemicals and tubing that lay on the back seat.

"What do you suppose would happen," I asked Bill, "if some crazed junkie decided to break into our car and steal that stuff?"

"He'd be in for a ride he hadn't anticipated."

"Well," I said, "better him than me."

We wandered to the downtown mall and chose a small restaurant, its windows adorned with wooden boxes holding bright tangles of pansies and petunias. Here we were served crisp, warm French bread and salads scattered with olives, feta cheese and sun-dried tomatoes. (I pushed some of the cheese to the side, guiltily savored a little of the rest of it—*pace* Dr. Lin!) A few doorways away, a trio of horn players, students at the Aspen Music Festival, filled the air with Mozart.

Finally, we made our way to the condo. Bill helped me bring in my luggage, we hugged each other hard and he left. None of my roommates had arrived yet, and I was alone with Theresa. I unpacked, setting everything—books, writing paper, underwear, clothes—carefully in its place. I noted with a small surge of relief that my room was adjoined by its own tiny bathroom: I was still self-conscious about my body, still half afraid even to touch it.

Within the next few hours, all my roommates convened. Celeste arrived, looking tan and healthy in her shorts and hiking boots, her glossy, straight brown hair falling about her face. Then came Mildred, a retired banker who was taking a travel writing course at the conference and who turned out to be wise, garrulous and able to drink like a trooper. Raylene from Kansas rounded out the quartet. She had very short, stylishly waved hair, long brown legs, clear, unlined skin and a smooth, kindly manner. For a couple of hours, we all sat around the table in the living room talking, sharing fruit Celeste had brought, speculating on the shape of the conference.

I was delighted with these roommates. I knew from past conferences that it was possible to be housed with neurotic, desperately lonely people. Or with a young, idealistic writer who'd want the two weeks of the workshop to take on the hush and exaltation of a religious retreat—the kind of person in front of whom you're embarrassed to switch on the television set, eat spare ribs or flip through a woman's magazine. But Celeste, Mildred and Raylene were so clearly tolerant and grown-up types that I found asking their permission to simmer vile-smelling herbs in the kitchen every morning quite easy. Their response was entirely reassuring.

Caryn McVoy, who was also attending the conference, arrived from her home in Carbondale. She, Celeste and I retired to my bedroom, where we spent an hour sprawled on the bed comparing notes about the last year. Caryn had gotten a short story accepted by a literary journal. One of Celeste's children's stories was about to come out as a book. I, too, had had a short story published. Feeling mildly triumphant—we had, after all, made a little progress since the last conference—we left for the introductory meeting at the Aspen Community Center.

There we checked out our fellow conferees. Almost all the men were bearded, and everyone was casually dressed. Tanned Aspen women in sleekly fitting blue jeans, long earrings, scarlet nail polish and T-shirts painted in swirls of primary colors mingled with carelessly dressed mountain types and drawn, intense women from New York, whose legs—dead white in baggy shorts—were clearly seeing their first sunshine in years.

I knew from past experience that you couldn't tell from appearances who the real writers were. The woman with the fiercely up-springing black curls, intelligent eyes and ironic smile would turn out to write flat, coy little stories about animals. The brooding young man who looked like James Dean would be the creator of pinkly pulsating romantic verses. But the fat woman who laughed too loudly and whose turquoise pantsuit exaggerated every unfortunate bulge would be a true poet whose spare, brilliantly evocative lines about boxing created new insights into the meaning of violence.

Writers attend conferences for a number of reasons: to break up the loneliness of those interminable hours in front of the computer, to befriend other writers, to get a serious evaluation of our work, to make contacts. But the biggest lure is the Famous Writer with whom we're assigned to study. We hope to gain inspiration from her simple proximity, perhaps to learn a few of her tricks. Most of all, we hope that, before the conference ends, she will have laid her cool hand on the brow of a favored one of us and said softly, "You have talent, my child. Go forth and write."

Most of the Famous Writers had come to the introductory session. Celeste located hers, novelist Joan Silber, at the end of the meeting, approached her and made herself known. She came back elated. "She seems wonderful," she whispered to us. "Really open and friendly."

Caryn's and my Famous Writer was nowhere to be seen. "I hope it's not an omen," muttered Caryn, "or that she didn't think her students were worth her time." After a few brief announcements, we all walked over to the Aspen Art Museum. Here, on a green patch of ground edging a little wood, conference organizers had set up a picnic.

Caryn, Celeste and I were sitting on the grass, sipping from paper cups of juice and picking at the fruits, salads and breads on our plates when someone said, "She's here."

I glanced across and felt a moment's misgiving. There stood a pale, slightly plump woman in a drooping light blue dress. Her hair hung straight. Her head was tilted a little to the side in a manner that looked—if such a thing were possible—at once sullen and coy. "I sure hope we made the right choice," I said to Caryn.

But at the next morning's workshop, the Famous Writer was animated and charming. She spoke brilliantly and fluidly through the entire session. Her passion for language was clear, and she mocked fiction that relied primarily on plot. "But how do you move forward if you don't have a plot?" someone asked her bravely. "It's a lily pad to lily pad kind of thing," the Famous Writer responded, laughing. I was charmed. Later, though, I wondered how she would react to the novel chapter I intended to bring into class for analysis. It was about life in a sixties commune and filled with action.

Aspen is only a few blocks long, so Caryn and I had little difficulty in finding Dr. Mink's office that afternoon. I needed to have my blood drawn and analyzed to see if the white blood count was sufficiently high for me to undergo chemotherapy. In Boulder, the blood analysis always took place right before the chemo drugs were administered, as Dr. Fleagle had the necessary apparatus in his office. But here it would take a day to get the results.

Dr. Mink's office was upstairs in a small, brick building. It was warm, wood-paneled, cozy. A young nurse took me into a back room, pricked my finger, and caught the blood in a tube. This seemed much easier to take, somehow, than the invasion of a needle into my vein.

The next morning found me in my customary vile, pre-chemotherapy mood. Trying to fortify myself for the ordeal ahead, I bought a package of wildflower seeds at a poky corner store, thinking to sow them over an unkempt patch of the garden when I got home. In class, the Famous Writer seemed a good bit less charming than before. We discussed the first chapter of a novel written by one of the students. It seemed pretty well done to me, though our instructor had several criticisms. Fair enough. But each criticism seemed to veer off into a discussion of a completely different way of telling the story or revealing the characters. Soon it became clear that our teacher was describing what she would have done with the material, rather than dealing with the student's actual work.

"Self-absorbed," I wrote in my notebook.

Right after the workshop, Caryn drove me back to Dr. Mink's office. After a brief wait, he appeared and led me into his examining room, where he pulled out and scanned Dr. Fleagle's letter and instructions. I had read the letter on the way up. It said I was a middle-aged white female with Stage II breast cancer. That was, I knew, worse than Stage I—which indicated no spread at all, and a hell of a lot better than Stage III or IV.

Dr. Mink was short, compact, with the tan skin of a dedicated skier stretched over bones so clearly defined that his face looked like a mask carved out of shining gold-brown mahogany. I had a lot of nervous questions for him. Had he dealt with many cancer patients? Did he know how to administer chemotherapy? Did he want to call Patti Kealiher for instructions on the sequence of chemicals and saline? "God," said Caryn after we'd left, "you sure were obnoxious." This compounded my anxiety. "I was? I didn't mean to be. Do you think he dislikes me?"

But Dr. Mink remained calm and pleasant. After a few minutes, he led me into another room and asked me to lie on his examining table with my left arm slightly elevated. I was used to receiving the drugs sitting up and had mixed feelings about my supine position. On the one hand, it made me feel nurtured and taken care of; on the other, invalided and helpless. I looked away while Dr. Mink pierced the vein at the crook of my arm, but his touch was gentle and the chemicals burned less than usual going in. I glanced at Caryn, standing behind me, holding my right hand at about the level of my shoulder. Her eyes were closed. I remembered that she had had to do this for her father when he was dying of cancer and was filled with gratitude for her willingness to relive such painful memories on my behalf.

I squeezed her hand. "This kind of chemo's not really bad," I told her. "It's pretty mild."

She opened her eyes. "Is that true?" she asked Dr. Mink.

His head was bent over my arm, and he sighed. "There's no such thing as a good chemo," he said. "But, yes, this is not one of the worst."

As always, I drew a quick breath of relief when the intrusive needle was withdrawn and the ball of cotton secured to my skin with a Band-Aid.

"In Boulder," I told Dr. Mink, "they use Band-Aids with Snoopy on them."

He smiled, "I'll have to get some in. Wait"—as I started to swing my legs down from the table—"lie still for a few more minutes."

Finally, he patted my shoulder. "See you next week."

I made out a check at the front desk, with the chalky taste of the drugs in my mouth, and Caryn led me to the car. I had hoped to have my routine after-chemo sleeping done by the time my friends were ready to leave for dinner, but I was still dozing when I heard them cluster at the door, getting ready to leave. I wanted to call out, "I'll come with you. I'll come, too. Wait for me," but I was too tired and woozy. Still, I felt terribly alone and abandoned as I heard the front door close behind them.

The chemotherapy became far more difficult to tolerate in Aspen. I'd been proud of the fact that, in Boulder, I'd been able to ignore the sickness it caused most of the time and had gone about my work and my daily routine. I had expected to surmount the nausea and fatigue even more successfully in Aspen, where I would be distracted by new surroundings, different friends, the stimulus of fellow writers and a writing workshop. Instead, I found myself more anxious and sick than usual. I thought this might be because of the altitude. When I asked Dr. Fleagle about it later, he said that although the drugs did not accumulate in the body, their effect was cumulative: each time I received them, my system was a little more worn down and out of phase than it had been for the previous infusion. I remembered Jeannie Fuller talking about "hitting the wall" in the middle of her chemotherapy routine.

At any rate, my system rebelled when I tried to add the Chinese herbs to the seething mixture in my gut. I'd stand at the sink with the glass of black liquid in my hand, shaking with the effort to gulp it down. Sometimes I succeeded. Sometimes, I managed at least a few swallows. Once or twice I simply tossed the mixture into the sink in a rage.

"I can't do it," I told Dr. Lin on the phone. "I can't get five cups down."

"Then drink less," she said. "Four cups OK. Even three. Try drink at least three."

But there were days when I couldn't drink any at all.

Being with Caryn and Celeste was a strong antidote to depression, however. On the second afternoon, we all decided to take a swim in the condo's small, sky-blue pool. "I think I'll be OK," I said. "I think the swimsuit covers my scar." That was the fear I could verbalize. The irrational fear I was really fighting was that somehow my insides would seep out through the incisions under my arm and on my breast, or that pool water would breach the integrity of my skin—my body seemed so horribly vulnerable to invasion these days.

Soon we were standing in the pool, up to our waists in water.

"OK," said Caryn, "let's see that terrible scar."

I pulled the bodice of the swimsuit down a couple of inches.

"Oh," she said, "that's not bad at all."

"No one would ever notice that," confirmed Celeste. "It's tiny. I thought it would be much bigger."

We were giggling like coeds in a dormitory comparing bra sizes at the mirror, and the joking and reassurance abruptly cut my fears down to size. Now my scar seemed small and banal, a cosmetic problem instead of the symbol of a vast, shapeless threat.

I moved away from Celeste and Caryn and started breast-stroking across the pool. The warm water slipped soothingly over my skin, over my breast. It felt like a healing and a benediction.

The conference took on its accustomed shape. After our regular morning workshops, we'd have lunch at one of Aspen's hip, charming little eateries. Or we'd sit on the mall benches, watching children place balloons on the row of miniature fountains in the middle of the street. As the jets of water rose and fell, so did the blue and yellow balloons, and the children shrieked with joy. There was music everywhere we went. The Aspen Music Festival was in full swing, and duos and trios graced doorways all along the mall.

But Aspen brought out the anarchist in me, too. Everything was so expensive, and the populace was so rich. Whether we stopped at an ice cream stand for a frozen yogurt or joined the line at a box office for a play, a tanned and slender woman in an elegantly tailored linen dress or a T-shirt hung with dozens of glittering charms and buttons was sure to step in front of us and raise an imperious, manicured hand for service. "The very rich are different from you and me," I'd quote to Caryn, adding, "they're a hell of a lot more insolent."

I began plotting a short story told from the point of view of a serial killer. I visualized him skulking in the doorways of the Aspen Mall at night, slipping silently into step behind one of these aerobicized, arrogant, carefully preserved women. I imagined how her smooth brown throat felt to him as he closed his hands around it.

Because rents in Aspen were astronomical, the character of the town was changing, I knew from the newspapers. The director of the Aspen Art Museum had left town because she couldn't find an affordable apartment. The future of the music festival, which annually brought devotees from Europe and all over America, was in doubt because there weren't enough reasonably priced rooms for the students. Even relatively affluent members of the middle class—dentists, college professors, architects—couldn't afford to live in Aspen. Nor could the poor, which meant that the people who waited tables, sold shoes and made up beds in motels generally fell into two categories. There were working-class folk who lived thirty or forty minutes away in Carbondale or Basalt and drove into Aspen every day. And there were flaky, unconcerned college kids, who crammed, dozens-strong, into condos and apartments and drifted from job to job.

I called home frequently. I learned that Anna had won first place in her ranking at a karate tournament; I gave her permission to wear a gauzy blouse of mine to a fancy restaurant she and her dad were going to with Arnie, Amy and Alanna. Every night, I read the story we'd be covering in the next day's workshop and fell asleep, clutching Theresa.

In the morning, the author would read his or her piece aloud, and then we would all critique it. It was unclear whether or not the Famous Writer was reading these offerings in advance: her comments appeared improvised. As the week progressed, some students commented that she had lost their stories; later I discovered that one of the stories I had sent in my application package was missing when she returned the package to me. One morning, she placed a sticky bran muffin on top of a student manuscript at her elbow, scattering crumbs.

Finally, it was my turn to present my writing. I was preceded by a tall, frighteningly intelligent woman who read a wonderful story about a ballet class. She made graceful shapes with her words, reminiscent of the rigorously precise, repetitive patterns of the class. I thought her story was brilliant and was a little intimidated at having to follow her.

Then I read my chapter. I hadn't read it aloud before, and it seemed to me that some of the rhythms of description and dialogue in it worked well.

"Would one of you like to comment?" said the Writer, glancing round the table with a tight smile. "Some of you might be more at home than I am with ... this kind of thing."

So she didn't like it. I braced myself. The discussion was going to be painful, but I would doubtless learn from it. I poised to take notes.

One student said he liked the conflicts I'd delineated; another said the dialogue was good. Then they looked to the instructor for confirmation.

"This," she said, "isn't writing."

She made some points about the way the characters should have related to each other, should have talked, should have behaved. But in the face of her blanket condemnation, they didn't seem to matter much.

We began walking back to the condo. Caryn's sympathy was almost palpable. But I was determined not to be crushed, to learn from the criticism, to retain my faith in myself as a writer.

"Everyone needs to get toughened up," I told Caryn. "Only it does seem a bit unfair to have cancer and this Famous Writer both in the same year."

As the workshop progressed, the instructor's tone softened a little. She was much kinder to the work of a few of the participants, in particular the creator of the ballet story. In her private session with me, she was friendly and open, praising some aspects of the piece I'd submitted in order to gain admittance to her class, advising me to write more about a particular character she found vivid. But I never really overcame the impression I'd acquired of her contempt for us and our work.

The organizers of the writers' conference had been working with the Aspen Repertory Company that year, and we had been encouraged to submit stories to the group. The director would then select a few of them for the company to act out, and we would gain valuable insights into how well our scenes and dialogue worked. I had sent a story about two women in prison: one a college student imprisoned by a judge who wanted to make an example of her for dealing cocaine, the other a mother who had abused and killed her three-year-old child. I was notified that this story had been selected. The company would stage a ten-minute segment of it.

We sat in the large, white tent that served as the theater and watched two brief scenes. Then the director announced my story. An actress stepped onto the stage. She was wearing sandals and a baggy, shapeless, gray-blue dress. Her skin was very white, her face almost expressionless. She slumped into a chair. I knew she must be playing the baby killer.

She began speaking in a flat, quiet voice. Within minutes the entire audience seemed to be leaning forward, avid to catch her every word. Her conviction and intensity were extraordinary.

And those words were mine—words I'd labored over months earlier, alone in my study:

"I dreamed last night that we was going to see her. We was going up that little, curvy street in that swank subdivision where those people live that had her. There's all these fancy cars there, parked kind of crooked because of the way the curbs are. It's one of them hot, blue, swimmy days, where everything looks flat like in a postcard, and all the hedges and fences and bigwheel bikes look like some kid outlined them in pencil. I can hear kids playing. ..."

She spoke with a terrible, stifled despair. I was barely breathing. It worked. The scene worked. I didn't know if it was because of my writing or her luminous talent, and it didn't matter because at this moment the two elements were inextricably fused. I wished she would go on reading forever. I wanted to know how the whole story would sound in her mouth.

When it was over, I approached the actress. Her name was Bonnie Brzezinski, she said. She was friendly and animated, completely unlike the drooping, passive character she'd just played. She said she loved the story, loved the role. But I was finding the conversation oddly disappointing. It took a couple of days before I realized why. This woman had been so intimate with my words, it came as a shock to realize that she was a complete stranger to me.

As I was leaving, the director of the Aspen Repertory Company touched my arm. He said that he would like to hold on to my story and possibly stage it in the fall as a one-act play. Would I agree to that?

I'd be involved with theater again. "Listen," I said, "you cast the lady I just watched as Susan, and you can do anything you want with that story."

The omnipresent nausea had receded. I floated down the road and home to supper.

159

13
THE WHITE QUEEN

A couple of weeks later, Bill and I went to retrieve Anna from Trojan Ranch, her summer camp. It consisted of a handful of wood cabins set among the fir-studded slopes around Gold Hill, about thirty minutes' drive from Boulder. We walked into Anna's cabin, which had the cool, damp, musty smell, the cluttered, improvised feel, of summer camps the world over. We were overjoyed at the prospect of seeing her again, but when Anna approached us, her face was streaked with tears. She didn't want to hug us. She didn't want to leave the camp, the horses, her counselor, her friends.

Wiping her eyes with the back of her hand, she insisted on saying goodbye to the animals before heading for home. She sprinted ahead of us, tanned and agile, looking like a cowgirl in her muddy boots, baggy shirt and blue jeans. But—instinctual, unthinking—she still completed a couple of grand jetés and a quick pirouette on her way down the path to the corral. Here the horses stood, patiently flicking away flies with their tails. A short distance away, a sow lay on her side with a gaggle of piglets grunting and pushing against her. We visited two female goats and their progeny. The black and white babies danced back and forth about the pen, ran at each other and skittered away stiff-legged, like playful puppies. Periodically, they pranced up for a quick pull at their mothers' hanging, oversized teats. "Their names are Bonnie and Clyde and Salt and Pepper," said Anna.

"I'm glad Dr. Lin's diet doesn't allow me much meat," I told Bill. "I can face all these critters without feeling guilty."

My arms ached for my daughter, but she was still keeping her distance, and I knew I shouldn't press the issue. It would take a while for the three of us to adjust to being together again.

"Last year, there was a goat whose tongue was too big for his mouth," Anna said. "It stuck out all the time, like this ... ," and she pushed the tip of a pink tongue through the corner of her lips.

All the way down the mountain in the car, while I feasted my eyes on her, she chattered about horses and singalongs and taking care of the animals. "We went on a hike by Glacier Lake," she said. "We slid down the glaciers on our ponchos. I ripped mine. For lunch we had a cheese sandwich, a peanut butter and jelly sandwich, an orange, two cookies and barbecued potato chips.

"And yesterday, yesterday, we rode into town, and we stopped at the store and bought Häagen-Dazs ice cream. We had vanilla and chocolate and strawberry and some kind of nut caramel crunch. We passed the cartons from hand to hand all the time we were riding our horses back. The caramel stuff was great. I had mainly the strawberry, though."

Anna had had a boyfriend for a couple of days, but then he'd gone off with someone else. "This other boy, David, he found a wild rabbit that was hurt and tried to bring it back to health. But it died the same afternoon the goats were born. So we had life and death on the same day."

Finally, we were home. As we walked into the house, she looked around and said, "This is so danged civilized."

"Bet you'll enjoy having a john you can flush," said Bill.

"Oh, yeah. And I can't wait to take a shower. We only got to have them twice a week."

A little later, she came into the living room, damp and fragrant, settled onto the sofa next to me, and cuddled up. "I missed you, Mommy."

Life settled into its normal track. I was having one small problem at work: I kept forgetting things. I'd be trying to write "The car accelerated," only the word "accelerate" would have flown right out of my head. "The car asserted ... ," I'd mutter. "Asterisk ... accident. ..." It was as if the term I wanted had fallen through a tiny black hole, an unexpected crevasse in my mind. I knew the brain was a likely target for breast cancer cells, and each time this happened, I'd feel a stab of fear.

161

I also had some idea that I should leave the job and concentrate on my own writing. I was motivated partly by the desire to write as much as possible while I still had time, partly by some half belief in the Siegel and LeShan formulas that said patients who were following their dreams survived longer. But I loved my job. The content of the features sections I supervised varied satisfyingly: I could work on an in-depth story about homelessness in Boulder one week, a frothy fashion layout the next. And I had a talented, cohesive and good-natured staff, whose support had helped me through the last few months.

After a great deal of thought, I decided that quitting the job would be foolish. But with the clarity of vision granted by the cancer, I decided to acknowledge that I was at the paper because I wanted to be, because I loved what I was doing and therefore should do it with a grateful and generous heart. Eventually, this decision would be modified. For the time being, it stood.

The cancer had also changed the way I went about things. I still worked hard, and as meticulously as possible, but I was no longer obsessed with the job. If my boss was critical, if one of my writers was unhappy with his salary and I couldn't get him a raise, if an error crept into one of the sections—well, in the great scheme of things, that was hardly worth getting upset about. Tears and anger should be saved for what mattered. While I hated the fear that had caused them, I cherished my newfound clarity and detachment.

At any rate, there was little point in setting aside more time for my own writing. I was having a great deal of trouble focusing on it. I felt sick most of the time, and whenever I went up to the study, turned on the computer and began work on my novel, the Famous Writer's words came, unbidden, into my mind: "This isn't writing."

I resumed my visits to Dr. Wood. He said that I shouldn't expect to be able to write a novel or to make any major life decisions while on chemotherapy. And I should look at the things I had accomplished.

"Think of the way you've dealt with this illness," he said. "Your family is together. Your marriage is very strong. Anna doesn't seem to be too traumatized."

It was his job, I knew, to build my self-confidence. Still, I listened hungrily.

"Bill and Anna have been very good to me, very patient with all my fears and complaining," I said.

"You've been generous with them. It's generous to share your feelings and let them know how to react. The families that get torn apart by this are the ones where the cancer patient just goes into a room and closes the door. Those families really suffer.

"And as for this constant need you have to do more things, and to do things better, it sounds like theism. It's having a god that's external, that's outside of yourself, instead of realizing that the godhead—if you want to call it that—is within."

I did want to call it that. "I can see the god in other people quite clearly," I said. "I just can't see it in me.

"You know, I'll listen to a piece of music, or read a really wonderful line of poetry, and I'll think, the world doesn't need me to write. I need to do it, but the world already has Shakespeare and Samuel Beckett and Graham Greene and Margaret Atwood and scores of magnificent writers and poets ..."

"When you respond to these people's art," said Dr. Wood, "it's because those things are in you. How else could you recognize the elegance of a phrase, or the shapeliness of a concerto, or the fire in a piece of poetry if those possibilities weren't in you? The part of you that recognizes and loves an artist's brilliance is akin to it.

"I'm not suggesting you could write as these people did. Only that you understand that.

"And as for what you've accomplished in the last few months, many people looking at your activities would be touched by them." He placed his fingers lightly on his chest as he said this.

Right after the cancer diagnosis, I had visited another therapist, recommended by John Day. I wanted someone to lead me through the relaxation and visualization exercises I had been reading about. This man had treated me with great gentleness and compassion, and I had sunk into his sympathy like someone pillowing into a down comforter. But ultimately, I had found his approach stifling. I thought of Claudio in *Measure for Measure*.

"Why givest thou me this shame?" he says, when his sister offers sympathy on his impending execution. "Thinkest thou I can a resolution find in flowery tenderness?"

Dr. Wood's whole approach was cooler, more detached. He never came too close or preempted my feelings. Instead, he seemed to lean back a little in his chair, creating a clear space between us. Into this space I'd hurl all my chaotic and conflicting thoughts. And, miraculously, they'd begin to take form.

He never shied away from painful truths. At an earlier session I had been cheerful and cocky, convinced I was well over the shock of learning I had cancer. I said, "You know how it was when I first came to you, back when I thought I was going to die ..."

Antonio Wood raised an eyebrow. "And now," he said, with exquisite politeness, "you are under the impression that you're not?"

I was living a therapeutic cliché: Dr. Wood reminded me irresistibly of my lost father—his dark hair and slender build, his enigmatic smile, his grave and unfailing courtesy toward his patients—even his foreignness, the fact that he, like my father, was a refugee. So when he said that word, *touched*, I felt tears come to my eyes. He was touched by me. I had touched him. And then he said the most wonderful thing yet. We were talking about dying, and he suddenly commented, "You might enjoy it."

"What?"

"You might enjoy dying. You do things with so much passion and curiosity. You'll probably die the same way."

I walked out in a daze. He had stood my fear on its head, and suddenly I felt free, filled with fierce joy. To enjoy one's death. If such a thing were possible, it would surely be the ultimate affirmation.

I dreamed I had some young plants. They were a tender pale green, the color of shot silk. I was trying to plant them in my cat's soft, cream-colored belly, and she kept scratching them out. I was frantic. It seemed so very important that they take root and flourish.

Through the long weeks of fall, I was continually nauseated, tired, angry and depressed. I still felt the constant fear, like a shabby gray mist between me and the world. But all the insights that had accompanied it—the realization of how profoundly I loved Bill, the passion for savoring every minute, the joy in Anna—seemed to ebb. Under the onslaught of everyday tensions and muddles, misunderstandings at work, squabbles at home (Anna was watching too much television; she wasn't reading books), my brain spun aimlessly round and round like a squirrel trapped in an exercise wheel. I had lost the great gift the cancer had given me, while retaining all the anguish and sorrow. "I'm sleepwalking again," I told Dr. Wood.

I decided to visit a fortune teller. In the last few months I'd found a lot of the safe demarcation lines I'd drawn around experience had dissolved. I was open to myriad beliefs and possibilities I'd simply dismissed as daft before. I had a faint memory of my mother saying that a fortune teller had foretold my father's death, and I did believe that such glimpses of the future were afforded to some people. I'd been given a name—Jan Main—and I called and set up an appointment. Torn between curiosity and skepticism, I actually canceled twice before driving to the busy shopping center where Jan Main had her office.

The building was set back a little; high walls surrounded an airy enclosed courtyard filled with greenery and light. I opened the door of an office and saw a young man at the front desk. I barely had time to give him my name before Jan Main was in the room. She looked like a regular businesswoman, black-haired, large-boned, dressed in a tidy red suit. As she opened the door of a back room, I envisaged a space hung with dark curtains, a round table with a crystal ball. But she led me into a perfectly ordinary office and sat me by a desk. Then she plopped down opposite me. I looked into her eyes. They were as dark as if they'd been scorched. She seized my hand, but she didn't turn it over and look at the lines on the palm as I'd expected. Instead, she held it in a strong, warm grip and began talking very fast. So there was no opportunity for her to glean snippets of fact about me from what I said or to receive intuitive messages from the way I sat or spoke.

"First of all," she said, "there's a lot of presence of humor in your hands. You're a very funny woman. And you're broad-minded, you

165

know, open to other people's ideas. You're curious what they're about." Her voice was precise and clear, her tone musical.

"But there's still a refinement that you take. It's not that there's a necessity for you to strap a backpack on and go trekking in the Himalayas looking for some answers, you know. You would much rather read about it."

This was so true that I gave a startled laugh. My curiosity about other people's lives and perceptions had taken me into all kinds of strange jobs; had had me conducting in-depth interviews with murderers, victims of violence, social workers, lawyers, artists, steelworkers, psychotics, scientists. It had dictated my twin career choices: acting and journalism. But I had never been physically adventurous.

"Even though you're open-minded, there are certain limits that you put on yourself for how to get your information. You don't limit other people as much as you do you. So, if I were to say, 'I'm going to the Himalayas, you know, to find out the truth of life,' you would say, 'Go for it. How wonderful. I'm not going, thank you very much.'

"In this lifetime, you have a challenge for yourself. You are to keep all promises that you make. It's very hard, too. That's a promise you made to yourself.

"You say that in previous lives you may have broken promises. And so in this lifetime you are to be good. So that's possibly part of the refinement and the self-limitation that I see. It seems kind of a heavy sentence that you might place upon yourself if you fail."

What followed was a mixture of insights that seemed so accurate that I could, indeed, believe Jan Main was reading my mind and comments that appeared way off the mark. She spoke a great deal about a child who was supposed to come to me—a child in the shape of a man, probably my husband, and whom I was supposed to heal. This didn't make much sense to me. Then there was something about a house; something about making a lot of money.

She did, however, peg my profession.

"The way you speak about yourself is that you were born with great verbal tendencies, you have abilities to speak and tell stories and

166

make people laugh. And there's something about making jokes when you're suffering that was taught to you as a child and you became so proficient at it you became almost famous for it ... a small fame, but nonetheless, fame. So still communication is one of your specialties. It tends to bring the people who are suffering up."

She seemed to be talking about my decision not to leave the paper and focus on my own writing when she said: "If you do not begin to do some of the things that you came to do—the communication, the writing, the uplifting of people who are in suffering states ...

"That was one of the promises that you made to yourself, that you would begin to share your experience of how to turn the unhappiness into happiness."

She said *happiness* oddly, very fast and emphatically, and with a kind of plosiveness on the *p*. It was the same with such words as *impossible* and *inseparable*.

Jan could have found out I was a writer easily enough, I supposed, since I worked at the local newspaper (although, as an editor, I seldom had my name in print). Still, she seemed so clear and so positive that it was hard not to be impressed.

Twice, Jan Main commented: "You really don't plan to share your experiences. You're planning to save it for some future life." But then she added, "You're here and you've got it and you've had the experiences, and doesn't it seem it would be a whole lot easier to do it now?"

Throughout the consultation, I waited to see if she would say anything about cancer. She did not. What she did say was, "Now I think that you've been stressed for the last couple of months. The stress is going away. Within the next two months, I see some stress leaving. Two months from now you will feel very buoyant. The stress seems like it's been going on for some time, but it's over a temporary issue apparently."

My chemotherapy regime would be over in two months.

Finally, I told her about the cancer, adding urgently, "Please don't tell me if you see anything too scary."

"I don't see you dying of this thing. You plan on at least another thirty years of life."

Still holding my hand between both of hers, she proceeded to tell me about my past lives. She said that Bill and I had been coupled three times before—and each time we had died laughing. "That's how it is when the two of you are together."

As for Anna, she was "very intelligent, knowledgeable in many areas of the spiritual path. She's been studying many lifetimes. She is planning to be enlightened in this lifetime. She was born with a very high sense of awareness, actually." This certainly seemed to fit.

"She calls her father something like a saint. Well, I don't know, it's probably not a saint, but she considers him something like a king. She calls him the king of the sea. They have strong karma. They've known each other many lives, and they've mostly lived by the ocean together."

When I left, I didn't know if I believed Jan Main was psychic or not. Still, I had always had one basic approach when it came to dealing with the inexplicable. I simply believed, specifically and precisely, those things it pleased or inspired me to believe. At the age of thirteen, for example, I'd decided to believe that Jesus had been born to a virgin, just as the Christians said, because the concept was beautiful to me—and nobody could prove that he hadn't. My favorite part of *Alice in Wonderland* was the White Queen's assertion that she made a habit of believing six impossible things daily before breakfast. So I decided to believe Jan Main. She had confirmed many of my inclinations and had made me feel calmer and more cheerful than I had for days.

"I don't know whether her fortune telling's for real or not," I told Bill that evening, "but I do know that she fully believes what she says." Curious, he rummaged in a drawer for a tape recorder and went into the bedroom to listen to the tape Jan had made of our session. He returned with a quizzical expression on his face: "She sure is right on the money about a lot of things."

The next day I was driving Anna to ballet. We were listening to Randy Travis singing "Always and Forever." "Hey," I said, apropos of nothing we'd been discussing, turning down the tape, "do you ever think of your father as the king of the sea?" I expected a

"What do you mean, Mom?" but she said matter-of-factly, "Oh, yeah. Sure. I see me and Dad living by the sea. Can we turn the music up again now?"

We had finished dinner on a Thursday night, on one of my off-chemo weeks. Bill was putting the dishes in the sink. I came into the kitchen, carrying my plate. "Avaunt," I cried, snatching up my gnawed corn cob and poking it at Bill's back. "Have at you." He grabbed his cob from the bowl containing organic garbage and turned on me, and we fenced until I sagged against the wall in giggles.

I went into the bedroom, took off my clothes and slid into bed. There was a bottle of oil on the headboard. Virginia Williams had had it blessed by her pastor and had given it to me. "You can rub it on your scar," she'd said, "or just dab it on the middle of your forehead." I poured a little into my hand and rubbed it over the scar on my breast. Then, with oily fingers, I began anointing the incision under my arm.

A lump.

An indisputable lump in the depths of my armpit. Something different from the bumps and puckerings that normally surround a healing cut. Again the profound hush, the sense that the earth had hesitated in its turning. Again, that nameless emotion that balanced equally between awe and fear. I sat motionless, my fingers on my death.

I found Bill in the living room and asked him to feel the lump. "I'm sure it's nothing," he said. "It's probably scar tissue."

Later I lay in the darkness while he slept, frantically attempting to tame this chaotic new element that had come into my life. The lump was very symmetrical, and it seemed to be in exactly the middle of the scar. I thought of the nine-day-long seeping of lymphatic fluid into the drain. That must be it, I decided. Some liquid must have accumulated where the mouth of the drain had been, and it was creating a smooth kind of cyst or blister there. I comforted myself and slept.

On Friday I called Dr. Day's office from work for an appointment. Then I sat, unhearing, through a meeting. I edited the same paragraph of a story about fall fashion over and over again. At around two, I left for Day's office.

At first he couldn't find the lump, and I felt a flicker of relief. I must have imagined it. But then he said, "Oh, yes, here it is."

"Could it be something caused by the drain?"

"No. But it could be a cyst. I'm going to have to take it out and look at it. If it is a cancer, it's a very superficial one—right on the surface."

Candis put her arm around my shoulders, then told me to sit by her while she recorded an appointment time for the new biopsy. Dr. Day came out of his office, said, "Let me just check something," and began feeling around my collarbones. Again that odd paradox: his touch comforted me, even though I knew perfectly well he was checking for lumps.

I had an appointment with Dr. Lin later that day, and I asked her to feel the lump. "Is it possible he leave something in there?" she asked. "Some cotton, maybe?" I said it seemed highly unlikely. "Is probably nothing, Julia, but is good he check it."

At least I didn't have to worry about whether this surgery would coincide with a menstrual period. Thanks to the chemotherapy, my periods had stopped. I had greeted their cessation with sadness. I remembered a schoolmate when we were about thirteen whispering to me, "I've had a visit from my friend," and me—ever literal—responding, "Oh, who?" Most of the names women gave their periods seemed silly to me—the curse, the visitor. But friend was OK. Indeed, my menstrual cycle had been a dear and trusted friend, a silent and constantly recurring assurance of my fertility. I had been so proud of the fact that my body persisted in menstruating through the first few months of chemotherapy treatment.

"It's really over now," I told Caryn on the phone. "That's it. No more periods."

"You're the only woman I know who'd actually feel bad about that," she responded.

In the context of a threat to my life, however, my grief over the coming of menopause was muted. A year or so later, I found that I had simply postponed feeling the full force of it. Kathryn Bernheimer became pregnant, and I was filled with envy as she navigated her glorious belly daily through the features department. I'd find tears coming to my eyes when I watched mothers with babies, even when I threw out the last, useless box of Tampax in the bathroom. I daydreamed constantly about Anna's babyhood, the tender weight of her small limbs in my hands, her soft, tousled hair as she slept, the nestling confidingness of her body against mine.

On Monday, Bill drove me to the medical center, and I realized there is a hierarchy of misery. Every Wednesday, as we sped toward my chemotherapy session, I wished that I was simply going to work. Editing the most twisted and difficult story, wading through mountains of inane press releases, attending hours-long and acrimonious meetings—all these duties seemed sheer pleasure compared to receiving the drugs. But now, as we drove along the familiar streets, I was wishing with all my heart that I was going to Dr. Fleagle's office for chemo, instead of to the nearby medical center for a biopsy.

Finally, I sat on a gurney, wearing a paper robe. The veins on the back of my hand had become hard and bumpy in reaction to the chemo, and when a nurse attempted to insert a needle into one of them, the tip went straight through the vein. She tried again. She was becoming flustered. As she struggled, Dr. Lombard, the anesthetist who had attended the lymph node dissection, came into the room and hugged me. "Here," she said to the nurse, "let me do that."

She injected some numbing agent into my hand before probing for the vein, which was a relief. But the needle still wouldn't penetrate properly. Then she tried the veins on the inside of my wrist a couple of times, with no success.

"I'm sorry," she said. "Here I came out to help, and look what I'm doing to you."

"It's OK." I needed a moment to catch my breath. "If you could just give me a sec ..."

Immediately, a kidney-shaped plastic tray appeared in front of me. I drew back, confused.

"Didn't you say you were going to be sick?" said the nurse.

171

Moments later, Dr. Lombard finally slipped the needle in.

I climbed onto the table in the operating room. "Was I this frightened last time?" I asked the operating room nurse.

"Yes," she said, "I think you were."

Dr. Lombard appeared by my side, as comforting and familiar as I remembered her from the node dissection. She fiddled with something above my head that connected with the needle in my hand. And like the sudden, exuberant uncoiling of a spring, my brain left its tight, miserable circling, and I was at peace.

Again the tugging and snipping, again the nurse holding my hand, stroking my hair. Only this time, I heard Dr. Day say clearly, "Oh, this is nothing. This is only scar tissue."

14
ORDINARY DAYS

I waited for the joyous relief, but it didn't come. Instead I worried ceaselessly until the report came from the lab. I reminded myself that Dr. Day had been right during the first biopsy, when he'd said the lump was malignant. So he must be right now, I thought, when he said that I was fine. But doctors did make mistakes. Suppose there were cancerous cells somewhere in the sample? What would happen next? A mastectomy? Stronger chemotherapies? I couldn't imagine dealing with more poisonous drugs than the ones I was on.

The lab confirmed Day's opinion. The lump had something to do with a fragment of stitch that had not dissolved properly and had caused an infection (which meant Dr. Lin had been partially right in asking if anything could have been left in the wound). Still, the depression I'd felt since finding it didn't lift. That lump had brought home to me a truth I'd been avoiding. Throughout my life, I'd always confronted crises with the sure knowledge that eventually they would be over. No matter how stressful or sorrowful the event, at some point I'd be able to patch together the pieces of my life again and begin the process of recovery. Any ability to endure that I'd acquired revolved around the words, "Hold on. This will pass." The phrase adults use with grieving children kept floating into my mind: "Hey, it's not the end of the world."

But this crisis of cancer would never be over, and it could mean the end of the world, at least for me. I would be in danger for the rest of my life. With some cancers, if the patient survives five years after diagnosis, he or she is pronounced cured. But most doctors don't use the word *cure* in speaking of breast cancer, that treacherous and unpredictable disease which can return after nine, ten, fifteen cancer-free years. I even heard a doctor say once that no one is cured of breast cancer: some women just manage to live with it for several decades.

The fear of recurrence is so intimate. It's like one of those stooped, shambling, Dickens characters. You can imagine this creature walking beside you, tugging with clammy hands on your sleeve, blowing decay-scented breath in your face, talking incessantly in a kind of smug, mumbling hiss—a self-chosen familiar who refuses to leave your side.

You can't take a vacation to get away from the fear, because it travels with you. You can find a suspicious lump, develop an inexplicable cough, an aching joint, a frightening headache in England or Austria, Hawaii or California as easily as at home. There is no safety anywhere.

The worst of it was the fact that Bill and I had been laughing and playing minutes before I found the lump. It was as if I had been punished for letting down my guard. I was also filled with fury because the biopsy had disrupted one of my precious, chemo-free weeks. I thought of the routine ecstasies of those weeks as my reward for enduring treatment.

I told Dr. Fleagle about the second biopsy on my next visit. "I'm sorry to hear it," he said, hand on my shoulder. "But you're all right now?"

Usually, with my doctors, I tried to be the ideal patient—brave and funny and understanding. At that moment, though, I didn't have the heart for it.

"No," I said. "What I learned is that I'll never be all right again. That the way I've been feeling the last week or two—that's it—that's the way it's going to be. The fear may go underground sometimes, but one way or another, it'll be there for the rest of my life. Whether that's a short time or a long one."

Usually loquacious, John Fleagle didn't say a word; he only nodded.

When Patti Kealiher came into the room, I showed her my wrist. It was surrounded by a bracelet of bruises where Dr. Lombard and the nurse had attempted to insert the needle before the biopsy.

"Hey, Juliet," Patti said. "If you ever need an injection, or blood taken again, call me. I'll come to wherever you are. I mean it. I'm not saying I can always hit it the first time, but I sure do know your veins pretty well by now."

Oddly that bracelet of bruises—that very little hurt—unleashed a flood of emotion in me. Clearly, I'd been keeping a lot in check in order to put on a rational and reasonably courageous front through the surgery and chemotherapy. It's as if it hadn't been safe to grieve consciously while undergoing the treatments, as though I needed all my energy simply to get by. But it was safe to sorrow for my black-and-blue wrist. "Look," I'd say, thrusting it toward a friend or co-worker, "look what happened to me." And I'd savor the expressions of sympathy that followed. I wanted to be babied. I wanted Bill to hold me and rock me and smooth my hair. "Oh," I wanted everyone to say, "oh, you poor, poor thing."

Cancer patients will tell you that the last weeks of treatment constitute a very difficult time. The friends and family who so freely offered love and support in the first month or two have all gone back about their business. But this is just about the point at which whatever gallantry and courage you summoned up to meet the diagnosis are wearing thin, and you're feeling weaker and sicker than ever before.

One afternoon, I went to pick up Anna at ballet class. It was a few minutes before the end, and the students were doing a series of exercises across the floor. Anna was the only child in the room, and she looked tiny beside the grown women dancing with her. Yet she was as disciplined, as absorbed in the movement, as they. When she saw me, a brief smile flickered across her face, and she continued her work.

On the way home, I told her I knew this had been a rough time for her and asked if she wanted to talk about it. "No," she said, in a flat, uncaring little voice. Would she like to talk to Lynn, then, or Louise, or even Dr. Wood?

"No."

We pulled into the driveway, and then she said suddenly that she'd been angry with me for getting cancer, angry with Daddy for not preventing it, angry with herself. She said God must be angry, too, because she'd prayed for all of us every night, and He'd still let this happen. Then she left the car. When I came into the house, I found her sitting in Bill's lap, sobbing.

But Anna wasn't generally lachrymose. Most of the time she seemed to be doing well. One day I walked into the lunchroom at work, where she was waiting for me to take her home. At the table with her was one of the business reporters, Julie Truck—a humorous, bright young woman. They had their heads together, and they were laughing uproariously. When they saw me, they giggled harder and went into a round of "Shall-we-tell-hers."

"OK," said Anna, deciding. "Me and Julie have figured out what to do with that obnoxious guy who's running the chemical business that's making all the pollution around where Linda lives. See, there's this boy in my class at school, and he's always farting." Her voice went up on "farting" as though she were asking a question. "Anyway, we're going to lock him and the chemical guy together in a closet."

"Appropriate," said Julie, smiling at me.

"We'll leave him there all day," said Anna. "Without a gas mask or anything. Don't you think that's a good idea, Mom?"

As the days wore on, my hair got thinner and thinner. Periodically, I'd catch sight of myself unexpectedly in a mirror and think I detected a bald patch. But then I'd look closer, and it would seem to vanish. Still, my hair was unquestionably sparse, and it had the fraying texture you associate with the hair of very old people. My eyebrows had grown fainter; even my pubic hair was thin.

"Do you think I should start wearing the wig?" I asked Kathryn Bernheimer one day at work.

She hedged: "It's up to you."

I turned to Cynthia Wahl. "Cynth, as a woman and a friend, tell me, is it time for the wig?"

Cynthia hesitated, too. "Well," she said, "as a woman and a friend, yes."

From that day on, I never left the house without the wig. It was less fun to wear this time around and felt hot and itchy on my head. But Mary Franks had been right: because I had worn it to a chorus of compliments when I didn't have to, it was much less disturbing to have to wear it now.

My premature menopause was bringing with it hot flashes. At first, I almost found them fun. They were a novelty. I associated the rush of hot blood to my face, the profuse sweating, with the flush that follows sex. I thought of the European girls I'd seen on a trip to the continent when I was sixteen. They were so much sexier than the buttoned-up English girls I'd grown up with. There was a pretty Swiss teenager I met in Austria. I remembered her at a party, how the damp curls stuck to her flushed forehead as she danced and how she plucked un-self-consciously at the undersleeves of her dress to allow the air to dry her perspiration. Hot, glowing, laughing, she was a magnet to all the Italian and Austrian boys in the room.

Now I thought of her periodically as I lifted the soaked hair from the back of my neck, fanned myself, pulled off my cardigan only to replace it minutes later. But I soon understood that this new phenomenon had nothing to do with being reckless and healthy and young. It was something that shouldn't be mentioned to others, something embarrassing. Hot flashes are ludicrous. They stamp you as barren and old. In our culture, there is nothing remotely sexy about a middle-aged woman having a hot flash.

It also seemed amusing to me, and later irritating, that simply touching Bill, snuggling against him at night, always seemed to bring one on. I'd fling myself away from him in a fever and toss off the covers.

"It's the yang energy," Dr. Lin explained. "His yang chi." As we talked, I started perspiring. "Oh," she said, teasing, "so you feel it even long-distance? Is OK. I feel it with my husband, too." She leaned toward me, and we laughed conspiratorially, like teenagers gossiping about sex.

The hot flashes followed their own capricious logic. I couldn't summon one up to help me through a cold wait for a bus, for instance, or prevent one because I was writing a check at the

177

supermarket and the beads of perspiration on my forehead might make me look like an amateur forger. The things did as they did, when they did.

With this premature menopause came some concerns I'd never had before: estrogen protects women from heart disease and osteoporosis. I soon found myself having earnest discussions with pharmacists about calcium supplements (Dr. Lin's diet allowed me very little milk and no cheese). I learned that some calcium pills were useless. A pill that did not dissolve in vinegar would have little activity in one's body. It took some trial and error, but eventually I found a brand that passed the test. I also tried to exercise more, since I'd read that weight-bearing exercise such as walking, jogging and lifting weights helps strengthen bones.

Periodically, Bill and I bickered over food. I was following my diet with the fervor of the newly converted. "Do you really think you should put butter on the asparagus and sour cream on the potato and eat a whole steak?" I'd say, peering over his shoulder as I carried the plate containing my pale piece of turkey breast surrounded by vegetables into the living room. Usually he responded good-humoredly; sometimes he'd explode, "Anna and I aren't going to eat that tasteless shit you eat."

Every now and then I'd sin: Bill would buy me a small box of bittersweet chocolates; I'd order a half cup of real coffee after a meal at a restaurant. The rigidity of my eating habits had one positive side: it made these little deviations from the diet indescribably delicious.

One night, I had a terrible dream. Anna was in a train. She was showing the conductor a photograph of me and telling him it was of her. This was the ultimate treachery, and told me, somehow, that she was extremely dangerous. Bill and I held her down, and I searched her roughly for the photograph.

As we struggled, I suddenly realized there was a passenger quietly watching us. "I was in here earlier," this woman said, "but I was driven away by the anger and sorrow among the three of you. It is almost palpable."

Now, however, she smiled and nodded, apparently unperturbed by the way Bill and I were handling Anna.

"She's very wild," I explained, afraid the passenger would think us abusive. "She has to be restrained."

Finally, Anna's hands and feet were secured, and she was dangling upside down from a rack attached to the ceiling of the railway car, snarling like a wild animal. I leafed through a stack of photographs and found one of a hideous creature, with oozing, green excrescences all over its face. I took it to Anna.

"Why are you showing me this?" she said.

She looked and sounded so like her normal sweet self that my heart twisted. But then I decided it was a trick.

I said, "Outside, you're beautiful. But inside you look like this." I thrust the picture at her and screamed, "You're ugly. Ugly. Ugly." Her face crumpled, but I couldn't stop. "You're evil and ugly and lying and wicked."

I was horrified when I woke up and—almost to cleanse myself—told Anna a little of my dream at breakfast.

"I had dreams, too," she responded. "In my dream I split into two people. One was good and one was evil. The evil side was kind of like a skeleton with bits of skin and stuff on it. The good side was me. Really me. But it was deaf ... the bad part and the good part had to talk in sign language."

I never did really understand my dream. But at one point, I was talking to Antonio Wood about my relationship with my own mother. "She was very strong, very controlling and very critical," I said. "I had to fight for my freedom like a wild cat." Suddenly the image of Anna, tied up and raging, flashed into my mind.

Another night I dreamed that I had a glorious head of hair. It cascaded to my shoulders in gentle, gleaming waves. But then I realized it wasn't my hair. It was Anna's. And when I looked in the mirror, my skin was as fresh and smooth as hers, and my cheek round and soft.

At best, aging can be difficult. I knew even before the cancer that I would never achieve all my youthful dreams, never play

Juliet or Portia or Ophelia or Rosalind. I was even too old for Cleopatra. Any novel I wrote now would, for better or worse, reflect a mature world view. The half-formed, wildly romantic prose I might have tossed into the world if I'd started writing in my twenties would never exist—a negligible loss for literature, but a real loss to me.

I would never have another baby.

Throughout my forties, I had mourned the passing of my youthful looks, grieved over wrinkles and thickenings and softenings; tried to maintain good health and energy through diet and exercise; found comfort in my continuing fertility. But the cancer diagnosis and the chemotherapy had put the aging process into fast forward. I had been thrown into menopause and, month by poisonous month, was becoming more fragile, more hollow.

One morning I looked into the mirror, allowing myself to really see my yellowish skin, tired, dull eyes and patches of chicken-down hair. I felt old and dried-up and immeasurably ugly. As I walked into the kitchen, Bill stopped me. He held me close against him, then ran his hands lovingly over my head. "Mmmmnnn," he said. "This is wonderful. I've never felt your skull so clearly before—all the bumps and hollows of it."

Sometimes I'd think, absently or urgently, about metastasis— if, when and where it might occur. Cancer is no respecter of will or dignity; it will do the unendurable, the unimaginable. It can take out an eye, close up your rectum, eliminate a limb, make an imbecile of you, wrench your head down onto your shoulder, break your back. I'd ponder the pros and cons of the four likeliest sites for a breast cancer metastasis: the lungs, liver, brain and bones. Maybe a recurrence in the lungs or liver would be the least horrifying, I'd think. At least that would bring quick death. But bone cancer, supposedly one of the most painful forms, does tend to allow the victim a couple of extra years of life. And I had discovered something most healthy people don't realize. Under almost any circumstances, the human animal desires to live. When a dying person begs for death, he or she is surely begging for a cessation of suffering, not of being. I suspected that, no

180

matter what, I would be greedy for every possible minute of existence. I wanted time. Time to be with Bill and time to be alone. Time to write. To learn or relearn languages, to travel, practice the piano, read. Most of all, I wanted time to see Anna grow up.

"Time, you old gypsyman, will you not stay?" says that wonderful, rickety-rack old rhyme. "Put up your caravan just for one day."

I'd play with these questions of spread as though the choice of a site were mine to make. But there was one possibility on which I couldn't allow my thoughts even to touch. Not my brain. Dear God. Please. No matter what, let me keep my mind. Let me keep my soul.

It was a magnificent fall. The heat lingered, the colors of the leaves flared fierce and bright, and then came a long, slow modulation into coolness. One morning, washing dishes, I watched through the kitchen window as McDuff and Petra played in the fallen leaves. McDuff ran on a slant, plumed tail flying like the feather in a cavalier's hat, a jaunty tilt to his hindquarters; Petra bounced up and down on all four feet, like a child's toy on springs. When they plunged into long grass, I'd see Petra's head and haunches rising and falling alternately, in a rocking horse motion. Periodically, the two dogs came together and seemed to kiss, open-mouthed. Then she'd come in low and nip at McDuff's legs, and he'd dance away sideways, coming back to mock-snap at the back of her neck.

Through the summer months, Bill and I had struggled to define what was most important to us. We took regular walks with the dogs. We visited friends more often. Bill began reading *Alice in Wonderland*—somehow he'd managed to get through an entire childhood without experiencing Lewis Carroll, Edward Lear, Hans Christian Anderson or Charles Kingsley. He was delighted by the humor and playfulness of both the Alice books, and we talked about them on one of our walks.

"The thing that intrigued me," he said, "was how you're going along and there's this whole logical pattern and it's all making sense, and then Lewis Carroll suddenly throws in a joker.

He changes the paradigm so there's a completely new reality and a real disconsonance between what happens in one moment and the next. And then the logic follows based on that new paradigm."

"I envy you being able to read it fresh," I said. "It must be so surprising."

"It's like the way Alice keeps growing and shrinking. When she's going up and down with the different pills and potions, she gets herself in worse and worse fixes, because she can't imagine or anticipate what the world is going to be like when she changes, or her ability to act in it then.

"In all the years I worked at the planning department in Jefferson County, I was trying to create models of the future. And if you just changed one variable, everything changed. That's kind of the way I organize my reality in my own life. The models are just constructs, but that's the only way I know how to function. So the book really spoke to me."

I said, "What I remember most was the stuff about definitions and naming things: how the pigeon sees Alice as a snake because her neck is long and she eats eggs, and the deer has no fear of Alice at all until it remembers its name. Once it knows it's a deer, it knows deer are afraid of human beings."

At night, I'd lie in the dark, holding Bill's upper arm between my hands as if it were a rope pulling me to safety. I'd think about the joys of the day, and how each moment we're given is a bright fleck of light on a black ocean of uncertainty. And I'd think about our love for each other.

When I was in my teens, almost all my efforts had gone into not being ordinary. I didn't want to have babies because, as I arrogantly told my mother, any cow can breed. I wanted to be singular, special. I planned to be a great actress, someone whose inspiration and artistry would change the tenor of her times. Now I understood just how ordinary I was. Ordinary enough to get something as banal as breast cancer. Ordinary enough to respond to it in exactly the same way as did thousands of other women. The fear, the thoughts of suicide and self-mutilation, the euphoria that followed surgery and routinely came again during the off-chemo weeks, all were common responses. Many cancer patients received the same loving support from their families, the same outpouring of affection and concern from their friends that I had experienced. A junior high school principal, beloved in the Boulder community, told me that all her students had gone outside at the time of her surgery. They had formed a circle around the school and joined hands, sending her a pure wave of love and strength.

So I was nothing special after all, nothing out of the ordinary. My emotions and perceptions were as common as dirt. But dirt, after all, is the medium that nourishes all life. At certain times, the world became transfigured, and through the ordinary—in the hands of mothers wiping ketchup from their toddlers' chins at McDonald's; in the whistling insouciance of a mechanic greasing a car; in Anna's gravely concentrated dancing—I could see the divine, as clear as day.

Most particularly, I saw it in my marriage. Here we were, Bill and I, settled and middle-aged, knowing each other's bathroom habits and smells, skin sagging, waistlines paunching, Bill's hair receding year by year. Hardly Romeo and Juliet, Antony and Cleopatra, Tristan and Isolde.

The Elizabethans thought of romantic love as a reflection of divine love, as having the power ultimately to guide the lover to God. Now I was viewing connubial love in somewhat the same way. It was a small, peaceful and lovely reflection, I came to believe, of a universal love that illumined the universe and shone through each and every one of us. Unless we chose to block it. So that, yes, fallible and ordinary and limited as Bill and I were, we were still, after all, great lovers.

Not that we didn't have our disagreements. Gunner was planning a hunting trip that fall, and Bill decided he would like to go with him. Everyone agreed it was a good idea: Bill deserved some kind of recreation after the steady support he'd provided for me and Anna over the long, difficult months of diagnosis and treatment. The trip was scheduled to coincide with an off-chemo fortnight, and I assured Bill that Anna and I would have no

183

trouble handling his absence. But as the time for him to leave came closer, I found myself getting more and more anxious. And then, on one of my visits to Dr. Fleagle, he found that my white blood count was too low, and chemotherapy would have to wait an extra week. This threw us off schedule. It meant that I would be on the drugs while Bill was gone.

I brooded over this. I remembered the fight we'd had the day before my surgery, Bill pulling back the covers of the bed and roaring at me, "Get up, goddammit. You're not just going to lie there and die." I knew he'd been afraid all along that I'd turn into someone passive and clinging and complaining, someone who would limit his life instead of being a partner in it. We had always given each other a lot of freedom; we'd taken trips separately on occasion; we'd pursued different interests, socialized with different groups of friends. It was manifestly fair for him to get a break from all the intense emotion of the year and go on a healing trip with an old and dear friend.

But I didn't want him to. Logically, I knew I could keep things going without him, but I was afraid. Suppose I found a lump, and he wasn't there to hold and reassure me? Suppose the next chemo made me unusually sick? I couldn't bear the thought of sliding into a cold bed at night without Bill's comforting back to press myself against.

"You'll be fine by yourself," said Dr. Wood, "and he deserves to be able to go."

"Bill," I finally said, as we sat in the living room. "I feel terrible about this, and I'd never do it normally, but I don't feel good about being on chemotherapy and you being away."

He'd been expecting it. "Fine," he said. "I'll call Gunner and cancel."

"Please don't be angry with me."

"I'm not angry."

But he was.

So, apparently, was Gunner. Lynn told me that on the phone a few days later. "He feels Bill let him down," she said. "And I was thinking about it. I thought, you know, if it was me, I'd want

Gunner to go. I think I'd want some time to myself, even if I were on chemo. When Gunner's gone, I really enjoy the privacy. I can put things in perspective, and I get things done I'd never get done otherwise."

Suddenly I was furious. "You have no idea how you'd feel if you were on chemo. No idea at all."

"You're right," she said, immediately contrite. "I don't."

Lynn had been my confidante, my dear, calm, wise friend, for a long time. I had expected understanding and easy, instant agreement. But this year we seemed to keep missing each other. During her mother's illness, I'd wanted so much to help her. Instead, within a week of Cecile's death, I'd found my own lump and become completely submerged in fear. And Lynn, the supreme comforter, hadn't been able to help me either, being filled with pain and grief herself.

We said affectionate goodbyes, but I hung up feeling betrayed. Everyone seemed to be telling me I should let Bill go. I supposed I should. But I wasn't going to. I couldn't.

15
PINE BOARDS AND STRAWBERRIES

As the chemotherapy treatments came closer and closer to ending, they became more and more difficult to endure. Freedom was so near, I could hardly bear to wait for it another second. When a session was delayed because my blood count was too low, the mixture of feelings was overwhelming—the leap of joy at not having to suffer the probing needle and the poisonous drugs that day, mixed with fury because the entire horrible business was being prolonged.

After I had my first injection of the last two-week series, I spent a sick, sullen week. At last, Bill took me in for the final treatment. As I walked into Dr. Fleagle's office and inhaled the familiar disinfectant smell, I was overcome by waves of nausea. I swallowed over and over as Patti Kealiher took my blood. "Do you want me to leave the needle in till we've run the analysis, or take it out and stick you again for the chemo?" she asked, as she did almost every time. As always, I had trouble deciding. I didn't like having a needle in my vein for the ten minutes or so it took to test my white blood count. On the other hand, scar tissue and hardening had made it so difficult to pierce my veins that I hated the idea of being stuck more than once.

"I know, I know," said Patti, laughing. "Why does she always ask me this? Why doesn't she just decide? OK, I'll take it out."

I went into the chemo room to wait. John Fleagle came in. "You must be feeling terrific," he said, "knowing this is the last time." He went on to tell me that he was sure I would be fine, that I'd been doing everything right, had tolerated the chemo well, had a very strong body. I wanted to respond to his kindness, but I was too busy trying not to vomit.

"Your blood count's fine," said Patti when she came in. "We can go ahead. Hey, your last chemo. Doesn't that feel great?"

The nausea became more insistent. Was I actually going to throw up right on the floor? There was another patient in the room. Her chemotherapy was being administered through a port in her neck—a technique doctors and nurses use when veins are too damaged or when the drugs must drip into the system slowly, over several hours. I figured this woman had problems of her own. She didn't need to smell my vomit.

"I'm sorry," I got out, "but I really do feel very sick."

"Hey, that's OK," said Patti. "Let me get you a pan."

She placed a small, green, kidney-shaped pan beside me. I still fought not to throw up. It was too embarrassing. Like defecating in public. I swallowed hard and managed to laugh.

"That thing's so small. Do people really hit it?"

"Well, not all of the time. Now just relax, and let me know when you're ready."

"You might as well go ahead."

Patti began the infusion and started telling me a joke as the liquids drained into my body:

"There was this couple, and one night the wife asked the husband, 'Honey, if I died, would you marry again?' He said, 'That's ridiculous. You're not going to die.' 'Yes,' she said, 'but just suppose I did. Would you?' 'OK,' he said, 'strictly hypothetically, let's say I would.'

"'Would you have her live here in the house with you?'

"'This is really dumb.'

"'Would you?'

"'OK. Yes.'"

The woman with the port was smiling. "I think you told me this one last time, Patti."

Patti chuckled and turned back to me. "So then the woman says, 'Would you give her my clothes?' And he says, kind of resigned, 'Yeah, I'd give her your clothes.' 'And my jewelry?' 'And your jewelry.' 'And my golf clubs?'

"'Of course not. She's left-handed.'"

187

The nausea subsided; I rubbed the skin around the needle tip as I felt the familiar burning sensation. Then Patti was securing a ball of cotton to the puncture with one of the Snoopy Band-Aids, and it was over.

A few minutes later, I found her in the hallway outside the examining rooms. "Patti, I have something for you." I handed her a box of chocolates and at the exact same moment saw the green-paper florist's cone in her hand. "And I have something for you."

It was a long-stemmed, crimson rose. I hugged Patti. I cried a little. But I still couldn't shake the cloud of sickness and ill temper. It accompanied me to the car and persisted, despite the rose's perfume, all the way home.

On my next visit, Dr. Fleagle recommended that I begin taking a drug called tamoxifen. This is a synthetic hormone. "You had an estrogen-receptive tumor," he said. "That means the cancer cells needed estrogen to grow. It's as if they had a kind of lock on the surface, and they're searching for a specific key, which is estrogen. Tamoxifen acts like the key. It locks into the cells, but then it immobilizes them—it's like a key that won't turn. So the cells might still be there, but if they can't grow, you don't have to worry about them. No one's exactly sure how tamoxifen works, but that's our best guess at the moment.

"There are almost no side effects. A few women get a rash, though that generally goes away. Some say it causes weight retention. I do have to tell you that one study showed a higher than expected incidence of uterine cancer in women who took tamoxifen. But that's never been duplicated, and its positive effects in preventing recurrence are proven."

He didn't say, though I learned it later, that the drug has a limited life. Eventually, estrogen-positive cells can learn to replicate themselves without the aid of estrogen.

A week later, I was having lunch with an old friend, science fiction writer Ed Bryant. Though I'm not usually a fan of the genre, I've always loved Ed's stories. In strong, shapely prose, he delineates a world that's filled with gray mists and barely comprehensible horror, where reality shifts before your eyes, fear rises from everyday events and death and suffering rule. The woman in the white Honda, stopped next to you at a red light, may be a practicing witch; the fraternity boys partying next door may be performing rites of unspeakable cruelty.

We sat over sour spinach soup and potato-filled dumplings in the Russian Cafe on the Pearl Street Mall and talked. Ed is a small man, who still has the long, straight hair and round spectacles I associate with the sixties. His voice is as deep and resonant as a Shakespearean actor's, and he wears a silver belt buckle shaped like a shark. Sharks figure prominently in some of Ed's pieces, including the story that won the first of his two Nebula awards. He is fond of sharks, given to saying that they are unfairly maligned. "Everyone's always ooohing and ahhhing about dolphins," he'd grumble. "They're not so noble. A dolphin will rape a wounded shark, you know. Why don't people talk about that?"

"I was sorry to hear about your cancer," he said. "I know how frightening it must be." He paused a moment. "Something like that happened to me recently. Not as bad, because it's not life threatening, but still ..."

Ed has a wonderful way of telling a story—so clear, orderly and expressive he seems to be reading to a wide-eyed child at bedtime. It was his storytelling voice I heard now, nuanced, detached.

"I was going out to buy books, and I had just parked my car. I got out, and all of a sudden I couldn't see. My right eye was filled with blood."

Ed has diabetes, and it seems this could cause the blood vessels in the eye to rupture. Laser surgery can sometimes save a sufferer's vision, and Ed was about to submit to a series of operations. But the danger of blindness—eventually, the disease tends to affect the other eye, too—was pressing and real.

"It's odd when you're sick," I said a few minutes later. "You feel like you've fallen into a separate world. Other people seem to be sleepwalking; you look at them and wonder at the things they're caring about, putting their energies into. And, in turn, they want to distance themselves from what's happening to you, to feel

189

it could never happen to them. They don't know how to talk to you, either."

"When they hear I have diabetes, people always say, 'Oh, yes, I had an uncle who had that, or a cousin,' and then I see a certain look come into their eyes, a kind of panic, as they remember that this story they've started telling doesn't exactly have a happy ending. Then they abruptly stop talking."

"I was with a group of people who were talking about someone who'd died," I said. "I asked them, 'What did he die of?' There was this long pause, and then someone muttered, 'Cancer.' It's as if they thought the idea that cancer could be fatal had never crossed my mind."

"Right," said Ed, laughing. "They didn't want to be the first to break it to you."

I couldn't tell how afraid he was. I wondered how he'd be able to write with no or impaired eyesight. I said, "It's odd to reach the age when serious illnesses, illnesses we associate with our parents, are happening to us."

I felt a strong pulse of understanding, camaraderie, between us. I remembered that nature writer Annie Dillard had once said she rarely saw a wild animal—a squirrel or rabbit or fox—that wasn't damaged in some way, that didn't have a jagged ear or torn tail or limb that showed evidence of having been broken and rehealed. Now it seemed to me this was true of human beings, too, as we aged. Ed and I had joined the army of the wounded, and there was a bond between us that the glossily intact could never understand.

These were difficult days. Several cancer patients had warned me that depression might come with the end of the chemotherapy. As unpleasant as the treatments were to tolerate, they said, they gave a sense of protection, a feeling that significant action was being taken against the disease. Without the frequent visits to the doctor, the reassuring interchange with him and the nurses, a patient often became frightened and adrift. Fortunately, one of QuaLife's three-day workshops had been planned for Boulder that December.

My hair was still very patchy, but I decided not to wear my wig to the workshop because it might get in the way of any physical work we did, and surely among cancer patients my appearance would be unremarkable.

I arrived at the community building where the workshop was being held. In the hallway was a table containing labels, crayons, scissors, glue, glitter and ribbons. Two or three people were working painstakingly with these materials.

"Go ahead and make your own name tag," said the woman behind the table. "Do it any way you want. Get creative."

I just chose a red pen and wrote my name in capitals. Then I proceeded to the main room, a little stiff, very conscious of my balding skull.

"So you're Juliet Wittman," said a tall woman with blonde hair and clear, delicate coloring, peering at my name tag. "We've talked on the phone. I'm Sara Wolfe." She hugged me. She was every bit as beautiful as Robert Dakota had indicated. "Welcome to QuaLife." As we talked, someone touched my head. I spun around. A slight woman with a huge, impish smile was standing behind me. She pulled gently on a wisp of my hair and said, "Yup. Oh, yes. I remember this stage."

I relaxed. Clearly she, too, was a patient. I examined her gray hair, which looked full, lustrous and healthy.

"I'm glad it's a stage. Sometimes I feel that I'm going to look like this forever."

"Oh, no," she said. "It feels like that, but in just a couple of months you'll see. My name's Molly, by the way."

Our intimacy was immediate and effortless.

We were asked to stand in a circle and to give our names and reasons for being at the workshop. Once the circle was formed, I saw Patti Kealiher chatting with someone I recognized as a nurse from the hospital. As the facilitator called on each of us in turn, I found the group was composed of patients, family members, the two nurses and a handful of therapists. There was also oncologist Paul Hamilton, who had founded QuaLife. A tall woman with reddish brown curls spoke.

"I came because I needed help," she said, "and QuaLife better be able to provide it. I just found out a couple of days ago that I have metastasis. It's in my bones. And I'd been feeling so well. I had no symptoms at all." Her face crumpled, and the man standing next to her took her in his arms.

What followed was a tapestry of lectures, songs, exercises and group discussion. We were led through guided meditations. At one point, I found myself lying on the floor while two or three people touched me and murmured soothing words I'd requested. The words were, "Let the healing come." Sara was one of the people in my group. When her turn came, the phrase she asked for was, "There is joy and purpose."

In the afternoon, Sara gave a workshop on journal writing. Her cancer had been diagnosed when she was in her twenties. She had just graduated from college with a master's in business and begun work on her first job. She lost that job and her insurance when her employers learned she was ill.

No one was exactly sure what kind of cancer Sara had, and she took her slides to experts: a breast cancer specialist on the East Coast, a lymphoma specialist on the West. The first told her what she had was definitely not breast cancer; it must be a lymphoma. The second said exactly the same thing, only in reverse. All the doctors were pessimistic about her chances of surviving. What she learned from the experience, Sara told us, was that doctors don't know everything. Also that sometimes you have to go forward without all the information you need. John Fleagle had concocted the chemotherapy that saved her life.

Sara suggested a couple of writing exercises. As she turned to write instructions on the blackboard, she said, "I don't really want to do this. I have a friend who was always raving about one of his classes at the university. It turned out he liked watching the teacher write on the board because when she did, her butt wiggled."

She went on to another point; she was talking seriously and persuasively, writing as she spoke. And all of a sudden, she twitched her backside at us.

The workshop was beautifully organized. A variety of healthy foods—nuts, fruits, herb teas and juices—were arrayed on one of the tables for all-day snacking. No sooner did we begin to feel stiff from too much sitting and listening than the organizers would propose a physical game or a relaxing stretch. Periodically, we all came together and sang loud, jubilant songs. Most of the information we were given, though clearly New Age flavored, seemed helpful and sensible.

Someone told a story about a man who was chased to the edge of a cliff by a savage tiger. Desperate to escape, he began climbing down. Then he realized there was a lion pacing on the ground below, waiting for him. He hesitated. Above him slavered the tiger; below him roared the lion. He saw a strawberry growing in a crevice close by his hand and picked it. It was the sweetest fruit he had ever tasted.

Even the bathroom breaks were interesting. For some reason, all the breast cancer patients consistently chose the same moment to visit the john. Our realization of this fact was accompanied by roars of laughter, and pretty soon all kinds of observations were being bartered at the mirror or shouted over the walls of the stalls:

"So have you started tamoxifen? What's it like? Are there any side effects?"

"Not really. The effects are pretty positive—you feel younger and healthier. Well, I have discovered a slight tendency to gain weight."

"I had a lumpectomy. How bad is a mastectomy? Does it hurt a lot?"

"No. The node dissection's the hardest part, and that would have been the same for you. There's a kind of bruised, heavy feeling where your breast was."

The tone was loud, intimate, hilarious. We sounded like girls in a dormitory, primping for a dance, comparing dates.

I arrived for the next morning's sessions full of enthusiasm and found that a man from an organization called Inspirations was speaking. This man was not only uttering the most insultingly obvious inanities, he was working the participants into a kind of call-response dynamic.

193

"So what is it we have to avoid?" he'd declaim. And obediently the audience would respond: "Self-doubt!"

"What is it?"

"Self-doubt!"

"And again."

"Self-doubt!"

And so on, ad nauseum.

I began to feel angry, upset and alienated. Everyone else in the room seemed to be fully absorbed and enthusiastic, nodding and smiling and roaring out answers.

"Wasn't he wonderful?" said someone later, during a break. It was Molly, the woman who had fingered my hair when I'd first walked into the workshop.

I hesitated. I really wanted to be part of this loving and responsive community. But truth won out.

"I hate it," I said. "I hate what he's doing. The manipulation and the yelling and the oversimplification." I stopped. Would Molly dislike me now? But she just put her arm through mine companionably as we walked back to the session and said simply, "I'm sorry it's not working for you."

All the declaiming and consensus-building was leading up to something. We were each given a smooth, square, pinewood board and told to write our worst fear on its pale surface. I wrote, "Dying of cancer." Then we were to put down the reason for our fear, what advantages derived from it, and why it was necessary to conquer it. "It cripples me," I wrote.

I knew what was coming. The man from Inspirations wanted us to smash those boards. He brought two people up from the audience to show us how it was done. One was Sara. She stepped up to the board as the man held it in front of him, took a deep breath and appeared to center herself. Then she broke the board with one clean stroke of the heel of her hand.

We were told to stand in several circles and practice the necessary moves, and our rehearsal was accompanied by more patter. We punched the air over and over, while the Inspirations man and his partner circled the room, correcting our movements.

"All right," said the man. "Is everybody ready?"

Patti Kealiher was standing next to me, flushed and sweaty. "I'm going to do it," she said. "I know I can do it."

As I so often had on this road, I found myself envying someone else's certainty. I was afraid I wouldn't be able to break the board and would end up looking foolish in front of this roomful of people. I also feared the way that failing might work on my imagination later—suggesting, on some superstitious level, that not conquering my fear would cause it to materialize. At the same time, part of me was coolly and cynically evaluating the techniques used to galvanize us into action.

Finally, four people stood at the front of the room, preparing to hold our pine boards out for us to break. We formed lines. The theme from *Chariots of Fire* was playing full volume on the tape recorder, and the excitement and anticipation in the room were almost tangible. I had a confused sensation of noise, movement, glowing faces, a crescendo of action. I was one of the first people to step forward and hand over my board. Someone slipped a turquoise bandana over my head, as if I were an athlete or a warrior going into battle.

I looked at the board. "Don't look at that," said the man holding it. "Look at me. Look into my eyes." He was solid and kindly looking, with a squarish face and honest, warm brown eyes. I took a deep breath, adopted the stance I'd been shown and slammed my hand into the board.

Nothing.

"Don't let your hand stop at the board; try and hit through it," said the man.

I tried again. Nothing. But I could have sworn I'd held myself exactly as instructed, struck just as I'd been told to. I'll never do it, I thought. But I tried again. Still nothing. I didn't know how many tries they allowed, but it was clear I wasn't going to succeed. I imagined the people in the line behind me must be getting impatient and prepared to slink away to the back of the room.

"Try again," said the man holding the board.

I had completely lost faith in the process, but I took the stance and struck. I was just starting to turn away, when I saw, as if in slow motion, a huge crack beginning at the top of the board and sliding down to bisect it cleanly.

"You did it," said the man. Suddenly I was in his arms, weeping for joy, and the people in the line were surging forward to hug me and pat my shoulders and murmur their congratulations.

I held the precious halves of the board to my chest and watched as the other participants stepped up for their turns. Almost everyone in the room broke his or her board; some, like Patti, on the first try, others after repeated attempts. For the very few people who failed, the Inspirations man had words of comfort: it was the effort that was important, that was healing, he said, not the actual breaking of the board.

I was wondering at what had taken place, at the abrupt dissolution of my estrangement and disbelief. It wasn't that I found the talk that had preceded the board shattering any more credible or reasonable than before. It was just that an undeniable surge of love and joy had propelled me into a stranger's arms and caused me to weep on his shoulder.

The lunch that followed was welcome. We filled our plates with a variety of foods—vegetarian lasagna, a beautiful salad of pear slices sprinkled with poppyseed—and broke into small groups to sit outside and eat. Patti Kealiher was in my group, and so was Dr. Paul Hamilton, who facilitated as we went around the circle, each of us in turn discussing our experiences. A man who was about to undergo chemotherapy asked if any of us knew where to get a good wig. Dr. Hamilton talked about a patient he'd had in Denver who always became very sick when he entered the hospital building. "Finally," said Dr. Hamilton, "we got into the habit of giving him his chemotherapy outside. He would come and sit under a big tree in front of the hospital, and the nurse would administer his drugs there."

"What about you?" he said to Patti, who up to now had said little. "How do you cope with the pressures of the job?"

Sometimes it was upsetting, said Patti, seeing so much illness and dying. Once, she had dreamed that she had leukemia and had woken in terror. The next day, she went to Dr. Fleagle. "If I ever get leukemia," she said, "will you take care of me?" He promised that he would.

"It must be hard," said Dr. Hamilton. I leaned forward to hear Patti's answer. I had often wondered how she kept her equanimity, her unfailing kindness and good humor when most of the people she saw every day would rather be almost anywhere than with her. In fact, the sight of her quite literally made many of us sick.

"Well," she said slowly, "I know people think being an oncological nurse is depressing, but I like working with cancer patients. They really know what's important and what isn't, and I learn from them."

Later, I interviewed Patti and found out more about her. She had wanted to be a nurse since she was little. When she graduated from nursing school, a job on the oncology floor of a local hospital was the only one available. Here, under the caring supervision of the head nurse, she'd learned "practical things like chemotherapy and blood work, but also the emotional things about families and dealing with disease."

After that, she joined John Fleagle's practice: "I was only out of school two years, and he was out one, and we just made it into something big and wonderful. Up to that time, there was only one oncologist in Boulder. John Fleagle came in and got tumor boards going—that's where a group of surgeons, oncologists, radiation therapists, psychologists, radiologists all get together and discuss new cases. I started up the only I Can Cope that's ever been in Boulder. It was because of John that we got the radiation center: He really fought hard for that, he and Norm Aarestad. We were pioneers in Boulder. I think before that, most people went to Denver for cancer care."

Patti had arrived on the job with a list of things she wanted: "I remember thinking, I'll never get all of this, and within six months I had everything. ... It was like, sometimes he didn't understand why I would need something, but if I asked for it, he'd trust me and get it for me."

It had been Patti's idea to give the patients roses when their courses of chemotherapy were over.

How did she deal with it when a patient died?

Patti was silent for several seconds. "Some of them mean more to you than others. Some of them just really tear your heart out because they were so important to you."

She began describing a woman who had had inflammatory breast cancer, which is almost inevitably fatal.

"She stuck it out for a good four years; she was just a stoic. She was around when I got married. She brought me flowers when I told her that I was engaged, and she came to my wedding and hand-made a garter for me to wear with my wedding dress. And through everything, she'd let me treat her and she'd let me teach her, but she also knew that she had firm control and if she didn't like something, she'd let me know.

"Her lungs filled up with fluid. She'd come in so short of breath, and we'd tap her lung—you know, John would put a needle into her lung and drain the fluid out, and the two of us would sit in the room with her, cracking jokes. She told the worst jokes. Dirty jokes. She used to tell about Sven and Inge.

"When she finally got seriously ill, I was very protective of her. When we referred her to hospice, she got a nurse that I didn't like, and I let them know it. They changed the nurse."

Patti had gone to visit this woman when she was dying. "She didn't recognize me. She didn't even recognize her husband. I almost wish I hadn't gone to see her, because she was so fun and wonderful, I hated to see that last scene."

But a house call to another dying patient was different, Patti said. "We all sat on her bed and just talked and cried and laughed. ..."

She paused again. "I feel so blessed to meet the people I meet in this."

Did she have a sense of what happened at the moment of death?

"I disagree with doctors on this one. The family wants to come in and be with the person at that last moment on earth, and the doctors will usually say, 'There's nothing magical. You don't need to be there.' And that's mostly to help the family get some rest and not feel guilty if they miss it.

"But I have been with people when they died, and there is something. ... It's like you share something very special with them. And I believe they know you're there till the very end. As a nurse, if I'm with the family, it's like I've created a new link with them. In the passing of their loved one, I've created a bond. I don't know. It's hard to explain. But it's something that they will remember for the rest of their lives, and I got to share it with them and help them through it."

Some people seemed to accept death, Patti said, while others "fight till the very end. They don't sleep. They wake up scared and crying. Their pain isn't controlled because they're so anxious and angry. They want to have chemotherapy till the very end, when you know it's not going to do anything. ...

"And that might be the one person the chemotherapy will help.

"I had a man who had prostate cancer when I first started with Dr. Fleagle. He was a hospice patient, which means you're expected to die within six months. Five years later, he was still around. Some people have the will to live and don't mind living with all the pain. I think some people are too ornery to give up."

Then she said very quietly, "But I'm not convinced it's really giving up."

She was skeptical about theories of a cancer personality. "I don't believe people cause their own cancer. I do believe you have some control, but I don't know how much. I think when you're dying, you can kind of pick your time. It's strategic. It's like, someone has sat with the dying person for the last sixteen days. They get up and get a cup of coffee, and the person dies then. Because he wanted to be alone? Because he didn't want that person to see it? I don't know. But I have seen it many times.

"I believe you can in some ways help yourself, but I've also seen people who truly, from the bottom of their hearts want to help themselves and can't. I can't explain that. I don't believe they have this underlying thing in them saying, really, I'd rather die."

199

Now, sitting on the grass with our lunches, a couple of us asked Dr. Hamilton about QuaLife's philosophy: Was the organization implying that the skills taught in these workshops, along with good habits and positive attitudes, could save our lives? "We're not promising that the things we suggest—diet, exercise, visualization, meditation, living life to the fullest—will add a day to anyone's lifespan," he said. "But we do promise that if you do these things, you will really be living up until the moment you die. And it may indeed be that these practices do have a healing effect. Nobody knows enough about it yet to say."

The afternoon's sessions were quieter than the morning's. They included a talk by a dancer who had had breast cancer ten years earlier, and who provided a slew of useful diet tips and facts.

The next day began with a trust exercise. It involved a guide leading a blindfolded participant through an obstacle course, and I was very nervous about it. When I was designated a guide, I felt a moment's relief—I wouldn't have to struggle through a muddy course unseeing. But then I started thinking about my very faulty sense of direction. Suppose I misled someone, got him or her lost on the course and made a complete and public fool of myself? Suppose someone actually got hurt because of my inept leading?

QuaLife people took us through the course. Our partners were to be wheeled across a deserted road in a wheelbarrow. Then they were to crawl through a drainage tunnel; climb a net made of knotted squares of rope into a small shed and leave the shed by climbing through a window; navigate a swaying bridge suspended from two wooden horses; walk across a seesaw; and make their way through a group of thick trees with face-whipping branches.

I was assigned my partner: Joyce, a therapist whom I had liked instinctively from the beginning of the weekend. She was a lithe, slender woman in her thirties, with a short, fashionable haircut and a wonderfully precise-featured and intelligent face. Her hand in mine, as we set out, was light and dry.

The QuaLife staffer walked over with the wheelbarrow, and I had to indicate to Joyce, without any words, that she was to step into it. It was the beginning of my learning a complete new vocabulary. I could try to pat, pull, even shove her into place, or I could take her hands and place them on the wheelbarrow so that she could learn its shape and her task for herself. Looking around, I saw that all the guides had different techniques. Some attempted to take complete control, some indicated what was ahead to their protégés and then stood back a little. All the blindfolded people learned differently, too, some clearly preferring one technique over another.

Joyce was a bit tentative about the wheelbarrow. Then came the muddy drainage pipe. She began crawling rapidly, and I crawled behind her, hands on her waist. Suddenly she stopped and gave a little scream. "I could have sworn I heard a rat," she said as we emerged.

I felt very protective, but at this point Joyce seemed almost completely to lose her need for me. It took only the smallest touch to send her moving confidently in the right direction, as swift and easy in her going as a dancer. No sooner had she felt the net between her fingers than she'd scaled it—so fast I couldn't climb it, too, but had to run around the shed to catch her and guide her through the window. She stepped lightly across the swaying bridge. At the other end a QuaLife staffer appeared and took her hand.

"You're changing partners," he told me.

I was distressed. What I had felt for Joyce as she moved with such grace and sureness through the course was something very like love. Why was this man taking her away from me? Had I done something wrong? Looking around, however, I realized that everyone was changing partners on this leg of the course.

My new partner clung to my arm; she seemed lumpy and heavy after Joyce. I soon found myself adopting different tactics with her, being altogether more watchful and concerned. But eventually we got into a rhythm, and she negotiated the seesaw and some barrels half submerged in mud with no problem. My last job was to lead her through the wooded area, vigilant to protect her from brambles and branches. Then we were on a clear, easy road and we half ran, half skipped back to the community center to join the others.

201

The red-headed woman with the bone metastasis was laughing.

"She's unbelievable," said her partner, the man who'd inquired about a wig in our lunch group. "She almost gave me a heart attack. We were going across that bridge—you know how it sways under you—and she just stopped and started jumping up and down. Jumping up and down and laughing like a bloody lunatic."

"It was great," said the woman, lighting a cigarette. She smiled fondly at the man, and they walked together into the house.

The exercise had been designed as a kind of metaphor for the patient-caretaker relationship, we were told later. In most cases the guides had been cancer patients, the people being led, helpers. So each group got a sense of how it felt to be the other. I thought of the odd, almost-love I'd felt for Joyce. "This seeing the sick endears them to us," Gerard Manley Hopkins once said. "Us, too, it endears."

"We wanted you to understand that sometimes a patient needs complete nurturance and protection, and other times he really needs for you to stand back and let him go it alone," Sara explained. "And we wanted patients to know how difficult it sometimes is making the right decisions when you're a caretaker."

This time, we each picked up a box lunch from the kitchen and ate alone. We then composed letters to ourselves about what we had learned on the weekend and wanted to remember. These were to be mailed to us a month later.

We all convened for a final song. Across the circle, Patti Kealiher was holding hands with the nurse from Boulder Community Hospital, singing full out. I was moved by her willingness to give up her weekend to be with us. I thought about her steadying hugs and her many words of comfort and reassurance over the past six months and felt the tears come into my throat.

We were each given a wine glass of apple cider with a strawberry in the bottom, to remind us to savor the moment. As we sipped, we watched a slide show of the weekend we'd just spent together. Afterward, there were fervent hugs and promises to stay in touch, and I left the building feeling strengthened and happy. Only one thing troubled me. One of the slides had been of me, just after I'd broken the board. My face was contorted under the turquoise headband; my head a variegated map of thin, fuzzy hair and balding spots. I looked hideous.

Bill made no objection that evening when I placed the broken board in a position of honor in our living room. He refrained from pointing out (as, I learned later, most of the female workshop participants' spouses had) that it is not particularly difficult to break a board when you strike along the grain. "I know this must seem silly to you, with the karate you've had and everything," I said, "but I never thought I could do anything like this."

"I think it's great," he responded. "You should take it to work and put it on your wall. Then if anyone messes with you, you can just say, 'Watch out. I broke that board with my bare hands.'"

The next week, I talked to Antonio Wood about the workshop.

"It bothered me a little, because my response seemed so shallow and predictable," I said. "I mean, to be manipulated by all that New Age stuff into feeling love—actual love—for people you've only just met."

"It is love," he said. "And it's quite real. Of course, it's situational. You may not like the same person at all if you spend more time with him and really get to know him or meet him in some other circumstance. But at the time that it's happening, it's real. And there's no need to denigrate or dishonor it. Take it for what it is."

16
RADIATION

In the months of uncertainty following my diagnosis, any discussion of future events had seemed dangerous. I'd say to Anna, "You can have that on your birthday," and feel the familiar gulf begin to yawn behind my breastbone as I confronted the possibility that I might not be around for that occasion. The word *Christmas* seemed particularly dangerous. So when the holiday season arrived, I was filled with joy. I'd made it. My family was intact. We had much to celebrate.

Anna was playing Clara in the Boulder Ballet Ensemble's *Nutcracker* that year, sharing the role with another talented young dancer, Hillary Umbaugh. She had been rehearsing every weekend and several nights a week for months. When the performance came, she seemed to me to fly through the part, dancing the pas de deux with the prince, with its lush, romantic music, so lightly and sweetly it brought tears to my eyes.

The second night was to end with a cast party. The dancers often gave each other little presents to celebrate the last night of a performance, and Anna wanted to do that, too. In the spring, the star of *Coppelia*, Ana Claire, had given Anna her bouquet after the performance. Anna had kept it, and the mummified roses had hung above her bed all year. Now she hit on the idea of giving Hillary and each of the party girls in the cast one of those roses. I thought about the faces of the other children when they were each presented with a very dead rose. I also knew what the gesture meant to Anna. I picked my words carefully.

"Sweetheart," I said, "it's a beautiful idea. But I'm afraid the other kids just might not understand."

"Yes, they will."

I told her to do whatever she thought was right and left her bedroom. Later, as she ran out the door to the car, I was relieved to see that the crumbling bouquet was not in her hand.

That night it was Hillary's turn to play Clara. She, too, danced beautifully. To our pleasure, the girls had managed to avoid hostility or rivalry through the entire rehearsal process, remaining good friends and helping each other learn the steps. Still, there was a storm of tears in the security of Anna's bedroom later that night, as she reacted both to the loss of the starring role and to the fact that this most exciting event of her year was over.

We spent Christmas Eve, as we did every year, with Lynn and Gunner, Louise and Steve and a few other friends. In deference to Gunner's Danish heritage, Lynn always prepared a huge roast pork dinner with candied potatoes and red cabbage. After dinner, we sat in the living room, sipping tea and watching as Gunner turned off all the lights and lit the dozens of white wax candles ornamenting their tall, sweeping fir tree. The branches also contained homemade decorations and woven paper baskets filled with candy. It was a family joke, retold annually, that one Christmas I had set my hair on fire, reaching greedily close to a candle for a basket of Licorice Allsorts.

Anna woke us at six on Christmas Day, and we all opened our presents. As always, thinking of my more austere British childhood, I made a few deprecating comments on the size of Anna's haul— she had video movies, video games, clothes, CDs, earrings and a stockingful of marzipan, chocolate, fruit and nuts. But secretly, I also delighted in our ability to afford those things for her. I had bought Bill a handsome bomber jacket that, in the way it combined the luxury of soft leather with a kind of street tough hoodiness, captured certain elements of his personality exactly. He gave me the strangest present yet: a bright, red and blue stuffed parrot accompanied by a gift certificate he'd made up on his computer. He had noticed my fascination with parrots, the way I'd stand by the parrot cages at the zoo whistling and clucking— the big, colorful birds cocking their heads curiously at me—until he and Anna pulled me away. The gift certificate said that after Christmas I could go out and buy a parrot of my own.

Later, I cooked a traditional feast: turkey, stuffing and gravy, green beans with almonds, salad and mashed potatoes for the three of us and Bill's parents, who had driven from Denver loaded down with presents. It was a joyous reunion. Bill's mother had had health problems over the past year, and we had all seen each other less frequently than usual.

New Year's Eve, oddly enough, found me as mopey and depressed as Christmas had found me jubilant. Steve and Louise hosted an intimate gathering: our family, Lynn and Gunner, John and Douchka, all four of our daughters. As we did every year, we read a list of the predictions we'd made the year previously. They ranged from the political through the personal to the trivial. Reading them, we saw that some had proved accurate or partially so: John had said that the Russians would leave Afghanistan in 1988; I had forecast revolution in Haiti. (We were deeply impressed a year later when we saw that Gunner had predicted the big California earthquake—until we realized that he predicted a California earthquake every year.)

Douchka had vowed to quit smoking in 1988; Dana had intended to get a new pen pal from China; Gunner had said he would get in shape and run the Bolder Boulder. Joy, Louise and Steve's daughter, instantly chimed in that she would, too, and so did I. "I'll walk it," said Douchka. "OK," said Steve. "I'll be there as well. Laughing at everyone here who tries to run or walk it."

"A spaceship will land in southern Colorado and pick up Shirley MacLaine," Lynn had said.

There was some bitterness in this recitation of last year's insights, too. Lynn had predicted that her mother's cancer would go into remission. Nobody had foreseen mine. "In all important aspects," Bill had said, on the night before what turned out to be the most unsettling year of our lives together, "next year will be better." Thinking about our cheerful blindness and the unchartable journey that lay ahead, I was afraid.

There was one prediction that drew a murmur of assent, however. "Next year," someone had said, "we'll all be with the people we love on New Year's Eve again."

It was time for our new predictions. Anna vowed to "eat less grease and fat and get all these white things off my tongue." Steve decided the Ayatollah Khomeini would "die and stay dead." Gunner said, "Juliet will have more hair." And Douchka again vowed to quit smoking. To a small chorus of groans, Louise said: "One of these girls will have a crush on some boy. And some father is going to get really uptight."

Steve videotaped our conversation and, after the toasts and hugs of midnight, played the tape back to us. Again, I was horrified by my image—the patchy, mannish haircut, the pinched, stern look on my face, the grayness about my mouth and eyes. By contrast, the other women looked beautiful—Douchka tossing her silky, straight hair, clear-eyed and youthful; Louise, an exotic, with a mist of dark hair and a piquant face dominated by huge, dark eyes; Lynn chatting, relaxed and sensual, her olive skin and black hair vivid against the oatmeal-colored sofa. These women seemed so alive, so sexy; by contrast, I felt like a ghost.

I had been given the holiday season off by Dr. Fleagle—a short period of respite before beginning radiation treatments. But early in January, I found myself at the radiation center to begin eight weeks of treatment.

The Miriam Hart Radiation Center was pretty new. Until a year or so earlier, when Boulderites needed radiation, they had traveled thirty miles into Denver to get it. Since radiation treatments are administered daily, this created some hardship for people who were very old or very ill. They had to find someone to drive them into Denver, as well as enduring the rigors of the journey. When Boulder's center opened, the staff found themselves treating far more patients than planners had predicted: clearly, faced with the transportation problem, many patients had simply decided to skip the radiation their doctors had prescribed.

The decor at the center was reasonably attractive. The rooms were decorated in a pinky-mushroom color—beige carpets, comfortable soft chairs—everything perhaps a little too muted and tasteful, but pleasant, nonetheless. Soft, formless music played continuously. On a low table in the waiting room were pots containing coffee and hot water, a bowl of candies and a variety of Celestial Seasonings herb teas. A faint, metallic smell permeated all the rooms.

There were current magazines in the racks, as well as a selection of leaflets and books, including a dear one written and illustrated by a nine-year-old boy who had survived a life-threatening bout with "cansur." He included a selection of advice to other children that was extraordinarily wise and stoical.

I knew that the radiation equipment itself was state of the art. And most of the staff, from receptionist Loretta Fox, a one-time breast cancer patient herself, through director Danny DeLange and medical director Norman Aarestad, turned out to be enthusiastic, helpful and compassionate.

I'd heard so many stories from cancer patients about visits to grimy, green-walled radiation rooms in the basements of large city hospitals that I was deeply grateful for the comforts of this building.

On my first visit, Loretta showed me to a small changing cubicle, where I replaced my silk shirt and my bra with a soft, much-laundered robe with three armholes.

"I can't figure out how to close this thing," I complained a few minutes later to Dr. Aarestad. "Do most of your patients have three arms?"

No doubt he heard that crack several times a day, but he smiled nonetheless. I was glad to see him again. I had fond memories of my first consultation with him, right after the diagnosis: his patience and humor, the clarity of his explanations, his elegant gestures, the remark he'd made about my upcoming surgery, "Have fun tomorrow."

He began explaining the purpose of the radiation. Sometimes there are stray cancer cells in a breast from which a tumor has been excised. The radiation is designed to kill those cells. In addition, cancer has a tendency to recur along a scar. For this reason, I would be given more intense radiation, focusing directly on the lumpectomy scar, during the last two weeks of the treatment. Some patients chose to have a radioactive implant for this part of the process, and that would speed things up; instead of coming to the center every working day for two weeks, I would spend three days in a hospital. The implant would be so radioactive that no visitors would be permitted to see me, however. Even the staff could not enter my room, but would slip plates of food through the door at mealtimes. It didn't sound appealing. And I didn't want my breast cut again. I chose to keep coming to the center for the last two weeks instead, and Dr. Aarestad assured me there was no difference between the two approaches in terms of effectiveness.

Would the radiation damage healthy tissue that it passed through? New techniques tended to be very specific and precise, minimizing damage, Dr. Aarestad pointed out.

Since I would be getting radiation to a relatively external part of the body, it was unlikely that I'd have a particularly adverse reaction: patients whose intestines are being irradiated can suffer nausea; those who are given radiation to the head and neck sometimes get headaches or become bald. I would feel more tired than usual, but that would be about it.

"When I went for the biopsy and for the chemo, I brought some music with me to listen to. Can I bring a tape here for the radiation?" I asked.

"Well, I'm not sure that you can," he responded. "I think they have some kind of radio that's piped in all over the building. Speakers in the wall kind of thing. Pretty ghastly music, too." He wrinkled his nose sympathetically. "But perhaps we could tune into a classical music station while you're here at least. Would that help?"

He handed me over to director Danny DeLange and bustled out. "I'll see if I can find a public radio station," he called from the door.

DeLange showed me into a room containing a huge, gray machine. I didn't look at it very closely, only lay down on a gurney as instructed and raised my right arm, placing my hand behind my head. DeLange began adjusting my position, propping me into place with wedges of foam. I heard the amorphous, treacly music change abruptly to Handel.

Periodically, as he fine-tuned my position and carefully adjusted my breast, DeLange would bring forward the huge mechanical arm of the machine, and sometimes I could see a silhouette of my breast and my nipple in one of its dark glass plates. He talked reassuringly throughout the procedure. Then he said, "I'm going to be pricking you eight times with a pin dipped in ink. It's like a tattoo. It'll mark your breast, so that the technicians will be able to focus the radiation."

"Will I be getting radiation today?"

"No," said DeLange. "I'll just be preparing you today. We'll start the treatments tomorrow."

Perhaps Dr. Aarestad had told me that. I couldn't remember. I felt the customary mix of feelings: elation at my reprieve, irritation that I wouldn't be getting at least the first session over with. Besides, I desperately wanted to know what radiation treatments would be like.

I tensed as Danny DeLange prepared the pin, but the prick didn't hurt very much. Only it seemed so odd to me, to be deliberately pricked on the breast. It's astonishing, once you've fallen into the land of the sick, I thought, the odd, offhandedly insulting things they can do to you.

Finally, Danny began marking my breast with a purple pen. He made Xs and some lines and asked me to try not to wash these off when I bathed or showered.

"I know you can't avoid the marks completely, and they'll fade a little," he said. "But do the best you can."

For the next eight weeks, my breast looked as if it had been bruised. The marker left purple stains on my white bras and was sometimes visible to the outside world if I wore an open-necked shirt. When the lines got too faint, one of the technicians would touch them up. "Is that what they pay you for?" I'd tease. "To draw on people with magic marker?"

"I didn't expect those pinpricks," I said, when DeLange was through. "But they really didn't hurt at all."

"Glad to hear you say that," he responded. "One woman told me they hurt worse than her surgery."

I felt smugly superior and told him that was ridiculous. But later I thought about how subjective pain is and how oversensitive the body becomes after surgery. I remembered how I'd shrunk from touch for two or three weeks, trembled at the prospect of even the smallest hurt. Louise, who's a psychologist, once told me that she had read about this phenomenon in a journal. It is physiological as well as psychological, the brain actually retaining some sort of physical trace of the traumatic event, which becomes activated at the threat of repetition.

I dressed and came out of the cubicle. The technicians, two young women, were watching on a video monitor as a patient received radiation. Curious about what I'd be undergoing the next day, I walked over. I caught a glimpse of a pair of legs sticking out of what looked like a tunnel.

"Hey," said one of the techs, whose name according to her name tag was Barb. "You're not supposed to be looking at the other patients."

"I'm not looking at the patient. I just want to get an idea of how the machine works."

"Well, you're not supposed to look."

She pulled out a black book. "We need to set a regular time for your appointment."

I had hoped to be able to get my treatments in the morning, leaving the rest of the day free for work, but there were no morning slots available. Barb filled in my name for three in the afternoon.

"Only I can't do that this Friday," I told her. "There's a two-day meeting in Denver I have to get to."

Irritably, she examined her book. "We'll get you in in the morning for that one day."

I was a little daunted. This was the person who'd be guiding me through the ordeal ahead, and we didn't seem to be off to a very good start.

The next day, Loretta greeted me and told me to go right in and change. I stripped to the waist in the narrow wooden cubicle, placed my clothes in a locker there, pulled on the three-armed robe and put the key, which was on an elastic band, around my wrist. Then I sat on a narrow bench to wait. I flipped through a copy of *Newsweek*. Barb had said I could keep my earrings on for the procedure, and I was grateful. The earrings—zigzagging green and purple snakes dotted with glass beads—gave me a sense of identity. I remembered how Carol at the medical center had allowed me to leave on my wedding ring through the surgery and had secured it to my finger with tape. When my mother had gone in for her colostomy, they'd taken off her ring. She said later that it made her feel like a corpse being stripped for burial.

"You're late," said Barb, coming to get me from the bench.

"I got here just a few minutes after three."

"Well, you have to be on time."

I couldn't afford her enmity. I said, "I'm sorry." But she didn't reply, leading the way into the radiation room. I thought with longing of Patti Kealiher.

I lay down on the metal gurney and positioned my right arm as Danny DeLange had shown me. My head was turned away from Barb. She slipped the foam pads into place to support the position, while I remained rigid. I understood that it was very important not to move. Then she pushed the gurney into place and adjusted the arm of the machine. I saw that someone had pasted a smiling raisin man, his huge blue-glove-clad hand raised in greeting, right at eye level—a small but significant touch of kindness. Beyond the machine, on the mushroom-colored wall, was a poster of a huge pinky-beige flower. Below that was a black box. I focused on the flower. The music being piped into the room was neither classical nor rock, but the kind of squishy mishmash some radio stations call "beautiful music" or "easy listening." I told myself I only had to hear it for a few minutes and that the people who worked here all and every day should have their choice of music. But a little Bach would have helped. Once, during a later session, as I lay staring at the flower, I suddenly heard Otis Redding singing "Dock of the Bay." It raised my spirits instantly.

Barb left, and I was alone in the room. The lights went down, and I saw a red beam shining from the black box. It bisected the shadow of my breast, visible on a glass plate. A whirring noise began. I knew Barb was manipulating the machine from the safety of her station outside the room. I knew that the room itself was encased in a foot of concrete: Gunner had told me once that he had driven by in his cab when the center was under construction and seen the buffer.

There was something unnerving about Barb's quiet, speedy exit. The machine was emitting beams so lethal that the staff—and, indeed, the entire population of Boulder—had to be protected from them. But all that terrifying radiation was being aimed directly at my right breast.

Some of my fears were less rational. I had visions of the machine getting jammed. I thought of Hiroshima, the moving figures burned into stillness on walls and sidewalks, black as shadows. But Dr. Aarestad had explained that the machine was programmed to turn off after the correct dosage had been administered, and, in addition, I was being monitored continuously by video.

The buzzing seemed to go on for a long time.

I tried to imagine the radiation as sun warming my body, gentle, yet strongly nurturing, burning away impurities, penetrating deep. I was not very successful. I took a few deep breaths and attempted to summon up some of the images from my most recent visualizations. I had been imagining skimming white birds flying through my system, picking cancer cells from the air as if they were insects. I delighted in the softness and warmth of the birds' feathers, the graceful patterns of their flight. But today they seemed sluggish. I feared that the radiation was doing them no good.

The machine stopped. Was the treatment over? I stayed absolutely still: Barb had told me not to move until told to. Suddenly I felt the gurney moving beneath me. I thought the machine was somehow being manipulated by remote control and was placing me in another position. I was too bewildered to realize that Barb had come back in, her white shoes soundless on the carpet, changed a glass plate and begun moving the gurney. Instead, as the movement seemed to falter at one point, I felt a flash of panic. I thought something had jammed.

The buzzing started again. I called the white birds in, and they huddled behind my breastbone, in the place where I imagined my thymus gland to be, heads beneath their wings. We waited. The buzzing stopped, the lights came up and a few seconds later, Barb came in. My right arm was stiff from the rigidity with which I'd held the required pose.

I dressed and went back to work.

The next day, as I sat on the bench, Barb deliberately called another patient in ahead of me—someone who had come in later. "Why wasn't I next?" I asked, when she finally called my name.

"You were late," she responded. "I told you not to be late."

I was nonplussed. Nobody at Dr. Fleagle's office had been punctilious about time. And I had made a particular effort because of our last encounter.

"I got here on the dot of ten."

"That's late. You were supposed to be in your gown and ready to go into the radiation room at ten."

Nobody had told me that. I lost patience. Clearly mildness and politeness weren't getting me anywhere with this woman.

"I see," I snapped. "So your calling that guy in ahead of me was punitive."

She led me into the room, adjusted my position on the gurney, redrew the marks on my breast, in cold silence.

The next Monday, as I changed, I heard a loud, angry, male voice. "I have to come here," it said, "and have these young girls fiddling with me. Wear this stupid robe and get fiddled with and put here and put there. It's not right. Why don't they have men getting us ready for radiation?"

I thought about the number of men who had handled my breast in the past year and smiled. This irate patient had a thing or two to learn. Then I walked to the bench. Someone had just gone into the radiation room, and the man whose voice I had heard was sitting by himself. He was ruddy and healthy looking, with dark gray, curly hair—and acutely uncomfortable in his short robe. He seemed unable to stop talking.

"Prostate cancer," he told me. "They found it last week. I was feeling perfectly fine, no symptoms or anything. Just went in for my regular checkup. And now they say I have cancer. But it might still be OK. They said I don't need surgery."

"How about chemotherapy?"

"Nope. Just this. This radiation stuff. Just a couple months. Then they think it'll be all right."

His eyes were feverish. In his hostility to the technicians, his nonstop babble, his unawareness of my existence as an independent being, I recognized the terror of the newly diagnosed.

"I just wasn't expecting it," he went on. "Cancer. Nobody in my family has cancer. They say this kind isn't the worst. They say it's slow-growing. I don't know."

I wanted to tell him that the acute phase passes, that life eventually continues in its accustomed paths after a cancer diagnosis. I said, "It's not so bad."

He responded, "Oh, I know. They told me. Doesn't hurt at all, they said. Not really something you feel."

Barb came out: "Mr. Burton."

"Good luck," I said.

When Barb came for me fifteen minutes later, I tensed. I wanted to be cool toward her. The more I'd thought about her officiousness, her obliviousness to her patients' fears, the more reprehensible I'd found them. On the other hand, I needed her to guide me through the treatments, and I'd be seeing her every day for several weeks. I didn't think I could afford her hostility. But she solved my dilemma, smiling pleasantly as she said, "Mrs. Wittman." I'd tell her later it was Ms., I decided.

Within a day or two, Mr. Burton had changed. He was now calm, friendly and avuncular. He began telling me about his family, about his mother, who was living in a nursing home. "It's a really nice one," he said. "We were worried at first about her going there, but this one's really nice. You can adjust the heat in your own room yourself, instead of waiting for someone to adjust it for the whole house. Gives her a sense of control."

He asked Barb about me once, she told me as she positioned me on the gurney. "He wanted to know what you had. He said it was a terrible shame for someone as young as you to have cancer."

I was touched, both by his ability to look beyond his own fears and empathize with mine and by the fact that he thought me young.

The process began to seem easier. "Gotta go," I'd yell, walking out of the features department at the newspaper. "Gotta get nuked." Barb became friendlier, and I began getting to know her partner, Kary Lewis. Kary was very slender, pale and pretty, with straight brown hair and thin white hands that were always icy cold on my breast. She talked to me about her boyfriend, whom she would soon be marrying. She told me that she had been working as a technician for several years, and in that time she had observed that the women coming for breast cancer treatments were younger and younger. In this, she echoed Mary Franks, the wig-fitter.

Did she think this was because cancers were being detected earlier?

"Maybe," she said, "but I don't think that would really account for all of it."

One morning both Barb and Kary were working on me.

"Mrs. Heiler finished up this morning," said Barb.

"Oh," said Kary. "So this was her last one?"

"She didn't want to be finished. She said she liked coming here—we're such nice young girls, and the doctor's so nice. 'There's nobody for me at home,' she said."

"Poor thing," said Kary. "Being sick and old and living all alone."

"We'll have to go visit her," said Barb, in a kinder tone than I had ever heard her use before.

Every week, on Wednesday, someone would take our blood. Like John Fleagle, Dr. Aarestad needed to be sure our white blood counts didn't drop too low to permit treatment. Mr. Burton and I joked with Barb and Kary about the thirsty vampires they must be keeping in the basement.

The blood was drawn by two different women who alternated weeks. As far as I could tell, they performed the simple procedure in exactly the same way. But while one of them slipped in the needle so deftly that I barely felt it, the other seemed to jab, sending a shock of pain up my arm. I always looked forward to the weeks when I saw the woman with the gentle touch.

A week or two into our treatments, Mr. Burton and I were joined on the bench by another man, an elderly Englishman with a loud voice and the kind of "haw-haw" accent—emanating, like a horse's neigh, from the nose and forehead—that I associate with P. G. Wodehouse characters: bluff old lords and blithering, oblivious colonialists. If Mr. Burton had been uncomfortable in his gown, this man was furiously so. He avoided our eyes, sat with his entire body turned away from us, pulled the pathetic little robe as far over his thighs as it would go and buried himself in a magazine. His feet—green-veined, oddly high-arched—smelled. I imagined the hard-sided black shoes that must usually imprison them.

Mr. Cronin, too, became more jovial as the days wore on, though he never really had much to say to me. He was very friendly with Barb and Kary, talking to them nonstop at the top of his booming voice. He also began a running dialogue with Mr. Burton, telling him about the small business he ran in Boulder, and how much better it was to work for oneself than for other people. If I said anything, he seemed to retreat. I thought he was embarrassed by me, perhaps by the nature of my illness, perhaps by the nature of his: like Mr. Burton, he had prostate cancer. Once I asked him where in England he was from. I wanted to tell him that I had grown up in London. He appeared offended at the question, however, and, after huffing and spluttering a bit, finally got out, "Of course I'm from England"—in a tone so like my old Latin teacher's that I fully expected him to add, "you stupid little girl."

One day, Mr. Cronin brought in a book by Dr. Seuss called *You're Only Old Once*. Here, in his inimitable blend of illustration and freely careering verse, the good doctor described a checkup at the Golden Years Clinic.

I had read *You're Only Old Once* before and found it an odd book. It's as good-humored as everything else by Dr. Seuss, and yet, as the shell-shocked protagonist reels from test to test, you can also sense the author's genuine fear. The book captures beautifully the way a patient becomes an object in the world of medicine, the inexplicable things that are done by doctors and technicians to the body, the concern that someday a test will yield a suspicious or threatening result.

Mr. Burton had never seen anything by Dr. Seuss before, and he was enchanted as he gazed at the brilliantly colored pictures: the goony, elastic-limbed figures, the amazing contraptions, the inventively shaped and proportioned hallways and rooms. He and Mr. Cronin sat side by side reading the book aloud to each other.

After all the radiation treatments were over, two images remained clear in my mind. One was of two old men sitting on a beige plastic bench, skinny legs pathetically vulnerable beneath their hospital gowns, roaring with laughter as—fluty British tones melding with midwestern accent—they chanted together:

"And you'll know,
once your necktie's
back under your chin ...
you're in pretty good shape
for the shape you are in!"

And myself lying on a gurney, surrounded by the huge arms of that gray machine, silent as someone enchanted or yet to be born; silent as a space traveler, encapsulated in metal and cast adrift in the black, reeling chasms of eternity; more alone than I had ever been in my life. Behind my breastbone, the white birds huddled, crooning softly into their wings.

17
LITTLE WHITE PILLS

The two-day workshop that disrupted my first week of radiation treatments was given by High Priority, a kind of publicity and education arm of the AMC Cancer Research Center in Lakewood. I had high expectations: this was where I had gone to Dr. Jennifer Caskey for a second opinion on chemotherapy.

Some weeks earlier, the High Priority director had called. She had told me that High Priority recruits women who are considered leaders in their communities to give workshops on the importance of regular breast examination. Over the two days we would be taught, among other things, how to do this.

"That'll be hard for me," I told her on the phone, "but probably a really good thing. I still can't bring myself to touch my breasts."

"Well, then, the workshop will be good for you, too," she said briskly. "You won't have any trouble after our video presentation and discussion."

So she didn't know I'd had breast cancer. "Aren't the women you're training patients?" I asked.

"Oh, no. Maybe some of them."

I hesitated. I had always thought this kind of organizing came best from those most affected. Still, I was flattered at being called a leader in my community and intrigued—cravenly perhaps—at the prospect of meeting the high-profile women who would be coming to the workshop.

The morning of the conference, I was scanning the wire at the newspaper when I saw the word "PILL" in capital letters. I called the story up on my screen. Three new studies had found a connection between the birth control pill and an increased incidence of breast cancer. As a result, a specially convened Food and Drug Administration panel was being asked by consumer advocates to require a warning label on all packages of pills. Reading, I was filled with a mixture of exultation and pure rage.

"I knew it," I said over the phone to Bill. "I knew I got breast cancer because of the damn pill. I mean, maybe I'd have gotten cancer eventually, given my family history. But I bet I wouldn't have got it in my forties. And millions of women have been on the pill. Remember all those people—Kary at the radiation center and Mary Franks, who sold me the wig—saying they were seeing patients coming in younger and younger? I'll bet that's the reason."

"Well, maybe it'll finally come out," said Bill. "Perhaps you can bring it up at the workshop and see what the doctors there say."

"Yeah. And it'll be great to be around some tough, angry women."

Though Dr. Fleagle had said there was no conclusive evidence of a link between my illness and the pill, my Chinese doctors simply seemed to accept the connection. "At least you know why it happened," said Michael Broffman, while Dr. Lin exclaimed, "That probably reason. Too much estrogen in body."

I had even tested the theory on the vet when I'd taken Petra in to have some suspicious lumps under her skin biopsied. "Lumps make me crazy because I've had breast cancer," I said. "But I think I got it from being on the birth control pill."

"That would do it," he said.

At lectures, I frequently heard doctors speak of the connection between estrogen and cancer. "Estrogen is the strongest promoter of tumors we know," said one. In a session at the local hospital, a well-known alternative healer wondered if there weren't some connection between the high incidence of breast cancer and the fact that more families were now eating chicken—frequently laced with hormones—in an effort to control their fat intake. But these experts seemed to shy away from making a direct connection between cancer and the pill.

I began taking the pill in 1964 at the age of twenty-two. I had just had an abortion. I was lucky: abortions were illegal in those days, but my abortionist was a medical doctor making a little money on the side. For five hundred dollars—very hard to come by at that time—he did a clean, thorough job and followed up with antibiotics and a couple of office visits. It was on the second of these visits that the topic of the pill came up.

"I wish that you had come to me sooner," he said, patting me on the shoulder. "I could have spared you all this trauma. There's a pill out now that prevents conception. Something new. It's really amazing, safe and effective. I wrote a prescription for my own daughter last week."

Soon I was carrying the pale purple Ortho-Novum package in my purse like a badge of honor, a symbol of how Bohemian and sexually free I was. Twenty-eight days a month I'd turn the plastic dial on the front, press out the pill beneath—the pills were so small you didn't really need water to swallow them—and gulp it down. I continued this procedure for seven years.

By the end of the sixties, I was living in a radical commune in San Diego, and I began hearing rumors about the pill. My housemates and I were inclined to be as suspicious of big business as of government, and we also tried to integrate healthful ways of buying and eating into our politics. This suited me well, as I had made a point of exercising and eating minimally processed foods all my life. I decided to stop taking the pill.

Soon after I'd made this decision, some of the women from the commune went to hear a presentation by feminist Roxanne Dunbar. I was very impressed with her. She was small and compact, filled with fierce energy, her hair close-cropped like Joan of Arc's. She was railing about available birth control options. She said, "And then there's the pill. My God, would any of us have taken it if we'd known it increased our chances of getting breast cancer by even the smallest margin?"

Increased our chances of getting breast cancer? That was something I hadn't heard from my kindly abortionist. But filled with the heady trust in my own immortality that all young people share, I wasn't particularly alarmed. I simply congratulated myself for having stopped taking the pill.

A few months later, the commune network was buzzing about a wonderful new contraceptive that had none of the pill's drawbacks because it didn't alter the functioning of the body in any systematic way, only placed a barrier at the mouth of the cervix. No one was exactly sure how this intrauterine device worked, since it wasn't solid and didn't prevent fertilization of the egg. It only somehow prevented the fertilized egg from being implanted in the uterus. The Lippes Loop, an older IUD, had been around for years, but it was so large that it was painful and impractical for childless women to wear. Now, however, there was a new version, a godsend for women like myself. In 1971, I had myself fitted for a Dalkon Shield.

My luck held. The only side effect I suffered from this dangerous device was menstrual cramping so severe that it sometimes doubled me over. Word on the hazards of the Dalkon Shield, however, hit the streets much faster than had rumors about the pill. I began hearing about women whose uteruses were perforated, who had suffered massive infections, who had given birth to full-term but dead or injured babies. There were some who lost organs and portions of organs to surgery because their shields had strayed; some who became sterile; a few who died.

By this time I had left the commune and was living in Boulder. I called the medical center. "I want an appointment with a gynecologist," I told the receptionist. "I want my Dalkon Shield out."

"Why?" she said.

It seemed doctors were telling women who were having no particular trouble with their shields simply to leave them in place. The reasons they gave were reassuring—"If it hasn't caused you any trouble so far, there's not much likelihood that it ever will"— but not entirely candid. The fact was that, having put Dalkon Shields into two or three million American women, the nation's gynecologists were having the darnedest time getting them out. Nasty little legged things, the shields sometimes traveled and tore a painful exit path for themselves, or had to be removed by surgery.

I was leading a charmed life, however. My shield popped out in seconds, without pain or complication.

"You must be really good," I told the doctor. "Some of my friends say it really hurt to get their Dalkon Shields removed."

"It's a simple procedure," he said. "There's no reason for pain or any other problem."

So I congratulated myself on being less of a crybaby than my friends. Until I met a woman who'd had a series of debilitating and difficult-to-diagnose ailments. By the time the doctors finally figured out what was causing her problems—her Dalkon Shield—she was forced to have her uterus, ovaries and part of her bladder removed. She was one of thousands of women who later sued A. H. Robins Co., manufacturer of the shield, but the same doctor who had told her in his examining room that her problems were caused by the Dalkon Shield refused to testify to it in court. Nevertheless, she, like many of the women who sued, won a settlement from the company.

In 1974, the device was taken off the market.

This experience caused many of us to distrust the medical system. One of the reasons I had never had a mammogram before I found the lump in my breast at the age of forty-six was fear. Could the radiation from a mammogram cause cancer? Was the medical establishment once again urging women to test an imperfectly designed product? I'll wait a few years, I told myself cannily, when I first heard the recommendation that all women should get mammograms, until all the kinks are ironed out, all the relevant facts known.

My caution served me as badly as my blind trust once had. If I had had a mammogram sooner, my cancer might have been detected while it was still microscopic and before it had spread to the lymph nodes.

So I arrived at the AMC Cancer Research Center filled with righteous indignation and in the pleased anticipation of acquiring more knowledge and perhaps some allies.

At lunch I met another cancer patient, Lynne Clampett. She was a nurse from a small town on the other side of the mountains, who wore the kind of permanently waved hairdo I associated with our mothers, a suit with a soft, pretty blouse, nylons and shiny black pumps.

We lined up together for lunch—a spread that included fish and chicken and looked both healthful and delicious. Unfortunately, Dr. Lin's diet allowed me none of the main dishes, and I had to fill my plate with salad and bread.

Lynne and I ate and talked. She had had two mastectomies, she told me, and her prognosis was not good; the cancer had already spread to the breastbone when it was discovered. She was cheerful and talkative, however, and she turned out to be a much freer spirit than her appearance indicated. Lynne had had no problem adjusting to a life without breasts.

"I like to hike and ride horses quite a bit, and who needs those things flap-flap-flapping in front?" she said. "The doctors suggested reconstruction or prostheses, but I didn't want to bother with them. This way I'm free. I feel like a ten-year-old boy."

Lynne's attitude was refreshing and unusual. Some women mourn the loss of their breasts for years.

"I had a ball when I went in for my wig when I was on chemo, too," she continued. "I made the girl bring out everything she had, and I tried them all on. I went home with one blond wig and one red one. That way I could dress up and go out at night and be whoever I wanted."

After lunch, we were shown to the hotel where we'd be spending the night and given time to unpack and relax. I discovered that I had forgotten to pack my tamoxifen.

"But that's all right, isn't it?" I asked Lynne when we all reconvened. "I'll just miss tonight's pill and tomorrow morning's and be back on the regime in the afternoon."

She hesitated. "It's doom," she said.

"What?"

"The way I understand it, it's dangerous to miss one. You know, if you have cancer cells in your body, the tamoxifen kind of stops them cold. But if it's not there, and just one cancer cell survives, that's it. You'll get a tumor somewhere else in your body."

I only half believed her. Surely Dr. Fleagle would have told me if regularity in taking the pill were that crucial. Still, I worried intermittently all afternoon. Later, I asked another nurse if it was OK to skip the tamoxifen once or twice, and she said comfortingly that she was sure it was. But it turned out she was speaking about medication in general and didn't know much about that specific drug.

I thought wildly about finding the nearest drugstore, calling Dr. Fleagle for an emergency prescription. In the end, I swallowed my fears and went on to the next part of the workshop.

That afternoon we were given information on what High Priority actually did. The organization created advertisements for glossy magazines that urged women to examine their breasts every month. Cher had appeared in one of these. There were also pale blue, plastic-coated cards containing detailed instructions for self-examination. These were distributed by High Priority for women to hang in their showers.

Then the director and her helpers showed us the videotape we'd be using when we gave workshops in self-examination to other women. It was very straightforward, honest and graphic. The woman who demonstrated the techniques was ordinary-looking, with reassuringly imperfect breasts, and the camera followed her fingers closely.

After this, a few rubber breasts made the rounds of the room. We were to palpate them, feeling for lumps. Each breast, we were told, contained several, each lump representing a different kind of cancer. Although there was something comical and obscene about these bright pink objects, the process of searching them for lumps seemed extremely useful to me, sensitizing our fingers and minds to what to look for.

These proceedings left me divided. I found the focus on breast examination and mammograms laudable: early detection was, I knew, the best hope for controlling the epidemic. But none of this did anything to help identify the cause of breast cancer or to protect women who already had the disease.

The director's talk was simplistic. She stated that, detected early, breast cancer is 95 percent curable. This, I knew, was not quite true. What was true was that a woman who found a very small tumor that turned out to be estrogen positive, well differentiated, diploid and dividing slowly and that had not yet invaded the lymph nodes—such a woman had an excellent chance for a long, healthy life. Though some of these women died, nonetheless. There were also some tumors that were so aggressive that they would metastasize, no matter at what point in their growth you discovered them, some kinds of breast cancer that had no cure.

High Priority's optimistic spiel, like the innumerable articles I'd read on early detection in women's magazines, was designed to convince us that vigilance and responsible behavior could protect us from untimely death. But nothing in life is that simple.

In addition, the relentless focus on individual responsibility meant that less attention was paid to other issues: basic research, carcinogens in the environment, the speed with which new drugs became available, the callous policies of insurance companies, poor women's access to care.

At one point, Lynne Clampett spoke up. She said that her tumor had not been palpable and had not been detected by a mammogram (mammograms miss 10 to 15 percent of breast cancers), even though it was large and had, in fact, already spread. "Well," said the High Priority director, cutting her off mid-sentence, "there's no need for us to talk about the times when it doesn't work. Most of the time it does."

A panel discussion followed, with several doctors available to answer questions. Center director Marvin Rich and his wife, Dr. Jean Hager-Rich—both of them short, stocky and talkative—presided.

Finally came the question I had been waiting for.

"Can you tell us more about the articles linking the birth control pill to breast cancer?" asked a woman in the audience.

A doctor on the panel responded. He said there was no proof of a connection, that the three studies the news stories had described contradicted dozens of previous studies. Their methodology was questionable, he added. And another problem concerned the validity of the data. Were the women being cited remembering accurately whether they'd taken the pill or not?

I began to tremble with rage. It sounded like the old myth about women being unreliable and hysterical again. I found it impossible to believe that any woman could have taken the birth control pill for any length of time and then completely forgotten about it.

The doctor continued, "It makes me angry that the media are unnecessarily frightening women. And taking the pill is less hazardous to your health than being pregnant."

"Right," I muttered to Lynne. "The only two choices available to women."

I didn't feel I knew enough to challenge the doctor on the spot. But I resolved to begin researching the issue as soon as I returned to work on the newspaper.

That evening we were given a magnificent meal, featuring wine, a whole variety of main dishes, dozens of cheeses and two full counters of dazzling desserts. Most of this was donated by local restaurants. But, remembering the quality of High Priority's printed materials, the sumptuous stationery, the fine lunch, I had to wonder how much of the AMC Cancer Research Center's resources was going toward research and how much to the kind of public relations activity I was witnessing. A well-known local photographer moved among the guests. This was no gathering of passionate angry activists. This was a society event.

One of the women at my table was describing her plan to bring a Grand Prix to the streets of Denver. I wanted to be polite, but I literally couldn't think of a response. I felt that I and my friends were fighting for our lives, while these people simply played around with the issues crucial to our survival. "You're talking about an actual car race?" I asked stupidly. "You're bringing a car race to Denver?"

At the other end of the table was the nurse who'd reassured me about the tamoxifen. I asked her what she thought of the latest stories on the pill, and she said, "Now I'm going to have dozens of patients coming in all anxious and upset. These stories just frighten women unnecessarily."

227

Again. "But maybe women should be frightened. Maybe this upsurge of breast cancer is frightening."

"There's no proven connection with the pill."

Dinner was followed with a presentation by a pretty red-haired young woman. She had constructed a sort of inspirational talk, filled with simple little aphorisms about how to conquer self-doubt. We were given a list of things we might be thinking—for example, "I can't do this" or "I don't have time"—and then provided with sayings to counter these notions. At the end of her speech, the crowd rose to its feet, laughing and applauding.

Back at the hotel, Lynne Clampett and I convened in her room. Lynne had a small plastic bottle in her hand. "Here," she said, "I just realized you didn't have to go without your tamoxifen. Let me give you a couple of mine."

I was filled with gratitude and went immediately to the buzzing hotel bathroom, where I poured a glass of water and swallowed a pill. Instantly, I felt safe, strong and happy. How odd, I thought, my assumption that this tiny white pill would so fully protect me. Wasn't my daily ingestion of tamoxifen, after all, uncomfortably reminiscent of the years and years I had spent faithfully taking birth control pills? And wasn't tamoxifen relatively new, its long-term effects unproven, the doctors unsure of exactly how it worked to deter cancer?

Later I heard there was a study linking tamoxifen with liver cancer; another that showed a correlation between the drug and eye problems. Yet most of the evidence indicated that tamoxifen did, indeed, delay recurrence. It also helped protect the heart and prevent bone loss. All in all, it seemed better to take it than to stop. At least this time my eyes were open. I remembered Sara Wolfe's observation that sometimes you had to go forward without all the information you needed.

But my mind only touched on all this as I settled comfortably on Lynne's bed for some late-night laughter and note comparing.

"My chemo was OK," Lynne was saying. "I could handle the nausea. But I hated the way I kept forgetting things—words would just pop right out of my head."

A great leap of joy almost stole my breath. "That's the chemo?"

"Chemo affects every cell that's dividing in your whole body. The cells of your brain divide, too, you know. So it's bound to affect your brain."

"I don't think my doctor mentioned that as a side effect."

"Those guys haven't been on chemo," said Lynne. "They don't know. Or they just don't think of it."

I was laughing, but close to tears. "Would you mind if I hugged you?"

She put her arms around me. "You thought you had a brain tumor, right?"

The next morning was spent organizing the women to lobby the state legislature for a very worthwhile new bill. It required insurance companies to cover the cost of mammograms and was later passed. I saw what the High Priority director had meant about community leaders. Woman after woman got to her feet: "I'll talk to the Board of Realtors"; "I've got friends at the Junior League." I racked my brain for an appropriate contact. Somehow, I didn't think my pre-newspaper association with the Committee in Solidarity with the People of El Salvador would cut much ice here.

Back in Boulder, I toyed with the idea of using the video, the pink rubber breasts, to give an early detection workshop to women at the newspaper or, on the newspaper's behalf, to the Boulder community. Early detection might have its limits and might not always be possible, but it indubitably saved lives. I didn't quite see, however, how I could reel off High Priority's cheerful canned spiel. I was also having doubts about the AMC Cancer Research Center's role in the world of cancer control, and I didn't want to be part of a glossy campaign designed to burnish its image.

Later I learned that serious inquiries were being made into the spending habits of Marvin Rich and Jean Hager-Rich. There were also questions raised about the percentage of the AMC Cancer Research Center's ten-million-dollar annual budget that actually went to cancer research. Soon after a long story about them appeared in *Westword*, a Denver weekly, the Riches left the center.

I began work on an article for the newspaper about the pill–cancer connection. I had found the response of the doctor on the center panel highly reminiscent of the obfuscatory dances I'd seen immediately after rumors of the Dalkon Shield's dangers had begun to surface. I soon found it wasn't that simple, however.

I called Rose Kushner, an outspoken advocate for women with breast cancer and author of *Why Me*, the definitive book on the subject up to that time. In her book, she had voiced her suspicions about the careless and ubiquitous use of estrogen.

"I'm going to be found out to be right," she said on the phone. "I've never wavered. Estrogen causes mammary tumors in five species of lab animals. If you want to grow a tumor in a mouse to see if a drug will work, the first thing you do is give it a shot of estrogen. It's the cheapest way to cause mammary carcinoma.

"Estrogen isn't believed to be the cause of tumors, but it promotes them, helps them grow. And in this culture we've exposed millions of women to outside estrogens—from hormones in beef and chicken to estrogen replacement therapy to the pill."

I didn't know it, but Kushner had suffered a recurrence and was severely ill. She died a few months later.

I contacted Public Citizen in Washington and received an exhaustively researched paper by Dr. Ida Helander. She analyzed thirteen studies reporting an association between use of the pill and breast cancer, particularly in pre-menopausal women. She also indicated that some of the studies that had previously seemed to show no connection, in fact did show a correlation when the variables were adjusted.

But then there was another study, this one on the effects of estrogen replacement therapy. It showed that women who took estrogen after menopause actually tended to live longer, because of the hormone's protective effect on bones and heart.

There's no real answer at present. It may be that tumors induced by oral contraceptives have a twenty- or thirty-year latency period, which means that discovery of a link is only now becoming possible. It may be that birth control pills are generally safe, but pose a danger to specific groups of women—those who have never been pregnant, for example, or those whose parents had cancer. Eventually, as DNA analysis moves forward, doctors may be able to determine who should or should not take oral contraceptives on the basis of a simple blood test.

Meanwhile, confusion reigns. All the studies that exist are retroactive, and some seem to contradict others: One finds a particular threat when the pill is given to teenage girls, another when it's taken by older women. In addition, since doctors began giving out the pill in the early sixties, it has changed. There is less estrogen in the pills women take now, and they often combine estrogen and progesterone, which may—or may not—reduce cancer risk.

The National Institutes of Health is undertaking a large study of the safety of oral contraceptives, using middle-aged women, both black and white. They will study five thousand women between the ages of forty and sixty-four with breast cancer against a control group of cancer-free subjects in search of a connection with the pill. They will also undertake tissue analysis. If the gene for breast cancer is found in the meantime, it will be folded into the study, according to a doctor working on the project. Data will be coordinated by the Centers for Disease Control.

So perhaps in six years' time we'll have some answers.

Lynne Clampett was one of the women who volunteered to test the birth control pill in Denver when it first came out. She had no doubt that it had caused her cancer.

18
SOUL HUNGER

The side effects of the radiation had not been profound. I was tired and a little depressed—both common complaints. On my breast, there was a slight redness under the constant purple marks, nothing more. Dr. Aarestad had given me an ointment, but I rarely applied it, still feeling a shock of pure terror almost every time my fingers brushed my breast.

One evening I found Anna in the bathroom, carefully mixing some liquid in a glass jar.

"I'm making a lotion," she said. "It's for you. To help where your breast is getting red. I put some oil and vitamin E and perfume in for you."

I hugged her. "Thank you. I know it'll help."

Bill and I were watching the news when the face of serial killer Ted Bundy came on the screen. It was a day or two before his execution, and he was talking to a fundamentalist Christian who had befriended him. He was saying that he had committed his hideous murders under the influence of pornography. Afterward, commentators speculated about his sincerity: was he just trying to ingratiate himself or somehow avoid the death penalty? But none of that had anything to do with what I had seen. Bundy's face had been pinched and yellow; I knew that his fear was a rank odor emanating from every pore. I could smell it. I had no sympathy for Ted Bundy. If ever anyone deserved the death penalty, it was he. But I tossed and turned in bed the entire night before his execution, linked to him by a primal bond of pure animal terror.

Mr. Burton and the Englishman both finished their treatments, but mine seemed to be going on forever. In the last two weeks, the machine was readjusted to give me a more concentrated

232

dose of radiation at the lumpectomy site. The beams made a dark and quite distinct red square on my breast.

"Oh," I'd mutter, slumped on the table, delaying getting into position. "I don't want to do this. I just don't."

"I don't blame you," Kary would respond, patting me into place with kind, icy little fingers.

Finally, it was all over. Two nights after the last treatment, I was stacking the dishwasher in the kitchen when I dropped a plate on the floor. It shattered. The next thing I knew, I was standing by the dishwasher positively keening with grief and rage, Bill was running from the back room to take me in his arms and Anna was standing in the kitchen doorway saying tremulously, "What's the matter? What's the matter with Mommy?"

Against Bill's chest, I finally said, "I broke a plate."

"Was it the crystal your mom gave you?"

I shook my head. Bill said, "It was just an old one, sweetheart."

I calmed down, hugged Anna and took her back to bed. I stayed with her for a few minutes, stroking her hair and neck in the dark, drawing comfort from her even as I gave it.

Later, I figured it out.

"It felt like I had to be calm and contained going through all the medical stuff," I said a few days later. "I couldn't really let myself think too much about what it was doing to my body—the surgery, chemotherapy and radiation—or what it was for. I kept it together and kept going to work and dealing with Anna nicely and calmly, and then it felt like suddenly everything came crashing down onto my shoulders, and I was thinking, My God, I had cancer. I had cancer. It really happened to me. That's what all those things were for. And I felt the full weight of the entire year all at once."

Bill and I decided to take a weekend off to celebrate the end of my treatments. Gunner had told us that many of his passengers talked about a local bed and breakfast called the Briar Rose. "They say they really take care of you there," he said. "They even have thick flannel robes for all the guests. One of the fares said that every day they bake fantastic butter cookies and serve them with tea."

It sounded ideal. I wanted to be cosseted. We arranged for Anna to spend the weekend with Gunner, Lynn and Dana and booked ourselves in for two nights.

The Briar Rose was a group of cottages tucked quietly behind a high hedge that bordered one of Boulder's busiest thoroughfares. The rooms were cozily furnished with old-fashioned wooden furniture, shelves of books, a scattering of ornaments and little dishes holding potpourris of dried flowers. On a china saucer on each bedstand was a single swirl of dark chocolate. And, to my delight, the bed itself was covered with a huge, puffy eiderdown exactly like the ones my parents had brought to London with them from Czechoslovakia and under which I had slept through all the years of my childhood. There was nothing like sleeping under pure goose down, I exulted to Bill—the softness, the way it drifts into place, cradling the contours of your body.

We went out to dinner. We made love under the beautiful comforter. We breakfasted on the feast provided by the Briar Rose: yogurt with granola, buttery little croissants with homemade strawberry and apricot jams. Giving myself a small holiday from Dr. Lin's restrictions, I sipped a cup of fragrant coffee.

Walking by the creek, we looked for signs of spring. Under last year's rustling, strawy grasses new growth was greening. Reddish brown catkins trembled on the alder branches, and the tops of the cottonwoods gleamed against the sky, their clear contour blurred by the swelling of buds on the topmost twigs.

At a special observatory built by the city, we watched the shadowy forms of trout slipping through dark water.

In the afternoon, we settled into the Briar Rose living room to read, and the owner brought out a tray containing a steaming pot of mint tea and a plate of the rich, warm-from-the-oven cookies Gunner had told us about.

"All these things seem to me so healing," I told Bill. "You know how you can get a really nutritious meal, but if you sort of wolf it down, thinking about your work or getting somewhere in a hurry, it seems like it doesn't really nourish you? Just knots up your stomach and doesn't get to the places in your body that need feeding? I don't know if that's true, but that's how it feels. Well, it kind of seems to me there're a lot of things like that. The trees budding down by the creek and sex and music and seeing Anna dance, and somehow I don't really let those things in. I don't realize them fully and allow them to nourish my spirit. Because I'm too busy or pissed about something—just plain not taking the time to be conscious."

"I feel that we finally are taking the time," Bill said. "We're doing more together, paying more attention to Anna. And—I know this sounds weird—you seem happier to me than you've been in a long time."

My first evening back home, I pulled out the seed catalogs I'd been saving as they arrived in the mail. I settled into an armchair and began perusing the familiar list from artichoke to zucchini.

I liked ordering seeds. I liked doing my part to maintain what I considered the ancient and honorable contract between gardener and seedsman. It's one of the few dignified, mutually respectful commercial transactions left. You don't see seedsmen creating flashy television commercials or empty slogans. They are much too busy nursing dozens of new varieties of plants in their search for that pest-resistant, juicily delicious tomato, or those huge golden-white marigolds. They know that gardeners can't be conned. Not for long, anyway. The tomato either resists pests or it doesn't; the marigold will not impress if it refuses to germinate.

Riffling the colorful pages, I imagined my completed list in the soil-stained hands of an ancient fellow at Burpee, Harris Seeds or Thompson & Morgan. He was wearing baggy gray pants held up with string.

"Hmmnnn," he'd mutter, "Silver Queen corn. Good choice. Good choice. Melody spinach. That'll do. Prolific anyway. Now what did she order those artichoke seeds for? It'd be hard for artichokes to do well in Colorado."

"I'll keep the plants well watered," I'd assure him. "And protect them through the winter. I think there's a chance I'll get some artichokes."

As I did every year, I ordered in two stages. First I went

through the catalog and ticked off every single variety of fruit and vegetable that took my fancy. Lettuce alone called for half a dozen check marks. There was looseleaf and butterhead; lettuce that came in red, bronze and varying shades of green; lettuce with leaves that were frilled, furled or shaped like oak leaves. The same array of choices existed for cucumbers. I could buy regular cukes; long, elegant European-style cukes; refreshing, lemon-flavored round cukes and little warty cukes intended for pickling.

I also put must-order marks by floating row covers, a pole arrangement for runner beans to climb, some plastic mulch and an aluminum hill arrangement for strawberries.

A few hours later, having given myself a serious lecture about the size of my bank account, the amount of space available for vegetables in the garden and precisely how much time I generally have for planting, watering, mulching, weeding, hoeing, controlling pests, and for pickling, canning, freezing, drying and making jam, I was back at the catalog, sadder and soberer, crossing things out. Few things in life were as pathetic, I reminded myself, as a gardener running around in early spring, a dozen bare-root strawberry plants in her hand, searching frantically for a fertile spot for a permanent bed.

The ordering finished, the envelopes stacked ready to mail, I lapsed into a sleep colored by visions of silver-green vines bearing clusters of pea pods; squash shaped like golden tennis balls; fragrant tomato vines; red potatoes nestled in black soil; armies of rustling corn stalks.

Ever since Christmas, Anna had been lobbying hard for a parrot. I was unsure, however, that I really had time to take care of another living creature. "You know, I don't groom Petra or walk her nearly as often as I should," I told Anna. "Heck, you and I don't even get to spend that much time together. I just don't think I could take on a parrot."

It was also hard to imagine how the bird would fit into our home. I imagined the cat gazing at his cage, stalking him continually. I thought with a shudder of what might happen were I to let a parrot fly free in the living room: one miscalculation, and the dogs would be on him and tear him to pieces. It seemed if we bought a bird, we'd have to keep him caged perennially in a little-used room, and I understood that parrots loved company and needed flight.

Finally, Bill and Anna inveigled me into visiting a pet shop. The selection of birds was not impressive—a few beautifully colored gray and yellow cockatiels, a green parrot, a bedraggled-looking cockatoo.

"That's Samantha," said the store clerk, indicating the cockatoo. We clustered round the bird's cage, and she cocked her head at us, then pulled herself upside down against the bars, showing off.

"We're selling her cheap," said the clerk. "Her people brought her in because they couldn't take care of her. They were away a lot, and it upset her so she started pulling out all her feathers. We figure she'll be fine if someone buys her who can pay her a lot of attention. ..."

Samantha let out an ear-punishing scream.

"They can get very attached to their owners," said the clerk.

I stroked Samantha's head with a crooked finger. I thought about the life spans of these big birds. Who knew how long I had to live? And even if I achieved a normal three-score and ten, I was now middle-aged, and parrots could live seventy-five years: I would have to will the bird to my daughter.

Anna looked back sadly as we walked out of the store. Samantha was plucking morosely on her shoulder feathers. "Maybe someday," Bill told her. "Sometime when Mommy can work at home."

A few days later, I was sitting in Antonio Wood's peaceful office, watching a squirrel scuttle about on his window sill. I said idly, "I don't seem to have much to say to you today."

"I think that's because you really don't need these sessions any more."

I stared at him.

"You're doing fine. You're a very healthy person. You don't need me any more."

The rational part of me knew he was right. I didn't need weekly therapy sessions. I didn't even know how long my insurance company would keep paying for them.

I tried to joke. "Hey, I could be unhealthy. Maybe I could work up some marital problems or something."

"I don't deal with marital problems."

I began to weep. Someone inside me was screaming, please Daddy, please Daddy, don't leave me again. I was furious with Antonio Wood, humiliated at my own lack of control and completely unable to stop the tears.

"Listen," he said. "I'll be here if you need me. You can call me any time. But you don't need regular sessions."

"If the cancer comes back?"

"I'll be here."

Eventually, I calmed down enough to ask if I could finish out the month. He agreed. As I rose to leave, he came over and put his arms around me.

"I know you'll be fine."

Ever since the diagnosis, I had felt a hunger for spiritual sustenance, for some truth-revealing vision, and now it intensified. When Virginia Williams again invited me to visit her church in Denver, I readily accepted.

I didn't really know what you wore to Virginia's church—I was pretty sure pants would be frowned on, but did I need to cover my hair? Or my hands? I finally selected a black skirt and white blouse. On the Thursday evening we'd agreed on, I watched as she came down the garden path to fetch me, picking her way carefully through the gravel in her high heels. She wore a cream-colored dress, trimmed and patterned in green. The formality of the dress made me see her differently: it accentuated the darkness of her skin, her slender grace. Her face was narrow, with clean, strong planes, her eyes quite literally almond-shaped.

In the car were Ginny's daughters: Connie, Vivian and six-year-old Melanie. They were all dressed up, too. Melanie, small for her age, wore a red and white dress with red shoes and carried a yellow plastic purse. Whenever I turned to look at her, she gave me a wide, impish smile.

As she drove, Ginny and I talked a little about our families. "Joe's very good with the children," she said. "I guess I do most of the taking care of them, but he's better at playing. He teases them. He has a good sense of humor."

I asked if all the worshippers at the church would be black, if they would mind my being among them.

"Most of them will be. But the church is for people of all colors."

"So it'll be OK for me to be there? And you'll guide me if I don't know what I'm supposed to do?"

She laughed. "All you have to do is praise the Lord. I'm sure you know how to do that."

"Oh," Connie cried from the back seat, amid a cascade of shrieks and giggles, "there's a bug. There's a huge bug." She pulled her legs up under her on the seat. "Get it away."

Melanie began half laughing, half crying with fear.

"Now where did it go?" said Vivian calmly.

"I see it. I see it," said Connie. "Help me smoosh it."

"I'm not going to help you smoosh it."

They bickered amiably all the way into Denver.

Because this was a state convention of the Church of God in Christ, a Pentacostal group, the service was being held in the ballroom of a hotel, instead of in the regular church. A plump, avuncular man shook everyone's hand as we entered. I was the only white person present, but he didn't hesitate when I came up to him, taking my hand in a firm grip and saying, "God bless you."

Connie and Vivian wandered off to join other teenagers; Ginny, Melanie and I found seats. Before sitting down, Ginny slipped to her knees, rested her elbows on the chair seat and prayed silently for a few seconds.

The room was cheerless, with drapes and carpeting in ugly shades of yellow and dully gleaming fluorescent lights. But the feeling in the room was electric, the worshippers gorgeously dressed. The men were in suits, the ushers in shining white gloves and the women resplendent.

A tall, thin woman wore a dress the glossy pink of the inside of a shell, her hair severely pulled back from her forehead and fixed in a knot with a multicolored pin. A plump woman had on a purple dress that was ruched, shirred and pleated around curves that gleamed proudly, sumptuously. There was a sprinkling of hats around the room—truly magnificent creations. A black lace fan was perched sideways on one woman's head; a black-and-white-striped whirligig adorned another's. There were also a number of tiny lace and flower confections.

The room was filled with children, all of them preternaturally tidy and well behaved: six-year-old boys in suits and ties and shiny shoes; little girls in frilly dresses and white stockings, their hair sectioned and decorated with ribbons or brightly colored barrettes. As the evening wore on, the children sagged quietly against their parents or leaned their heads against the backs of their chairs and slept.

A tall man strode to the microphone, half singing, half speaking, calling out slowly and passionately about God and Jesus and his need for them. Scattered cries of "Amen" and "I need you Jesus" answered him. He picked up in speed and rhythm, and the scattered cries coalesced like droplets of mercury. Within minutes, all the worshippers were on their feet, singing, clapping, waving their hands in the air.

Ginny had explained that this was a spirit-led church. Very little had been pre-set. People at the microphone spoke as their hearts dictated; the audience responded in kind. A skinny, bearded man stepped onto the podium, saying he wanted to sing a song that had come into his mind recently. He sang, "You're my rock, you're my fortress, you're my deliverance, in you will I trust." After a repetition or two, we all sang along with him.

Another speaker, a plump, elderly woman in a bright yellow suit, spoke of the joy in her soul and of wanting to fling her hat into the air. The audience clapped; several of them raised their open hands and shook them; and she began dancing in place on the podium, a kind of trancelike, holy dance.

Worshippers came and went during the service. Some people knelt, as Ginny had, before sitting down. A man standing near us shook a tambourine. I heard Ginny's clear, soft voice at my side, singing, chanting, calling on the Lord.

This was not the austere deity of the churches I'd visited before, but someone warm and real, almost palpable in the room. The worshippers were addressed as saints, and they all seemed profoundly at home with their God. "Give the Lord a hand," a preacher said, to thunderous applause. Another exulted, "He's all right with me. He's so all right with me that I brought Him with me. I bring Him everywhere with me."

A thin, angular woman took the podium. I had noticed her before in the crowd: she had been clapping, singing and swaying with ferocious intensity.

"We are at war," she said. "We are at war with the devil. I have statistics that tell us that immorality in the school has increased since prayer was shut out, prayer was excluded. Within six months, immorality had gone up fifty percent. By now it's up five hundred percent. It had to happen. It had to happen. Because where God is not, the other will be. Satan will be. He is filled with hate and rage. We must be ready to make war on him every moment and at all times."

Melanie slipped a lemon drop into my hand. "You want a candy?" She leaned against me, her eyes drifting shut.

Two girls of about ten came up to the microphone, accompanied by a third who seemed to be in her early teens. There was silence for a few seconds—startling after all the singing and oratory. Then a small voice began singing, "I know Jesus, I know Jesus. Do you know him, too?" The second little girl joined in; the teenager began humming an accompaniment.

I began to understand why the people came here so gladly. Time and again, a speaker called out, there were scattered responses, a woman stood up, clapping, followed by another. Around the room, whole groups of people rose to their feet. A drumbeat started, then the passionate whine of an organ. Finally, the cries, stamps, claps and chants merged into a great, crashing wall of sound and exultation.

If I was self-conscious at first, listening intently, folding my hands demurely in my lap or finding a place for them on the back of the chair in front of me, within minutes I, too, was swaying and singing. In deference to my Jewish heritage, I called on the Lord rather than on Jesus. And I knew that some of the politics of this church were probably not for me. But if I was a sort of intruder in this worshipful crowd, I was wholeheartedly part of the overwhelming emotion of the moment.

After a couple of hours, the congregation's energy seemed spent. There was some administrative business, some talk of district missionaries and first ladies and pastors and the state bishop. I began to glimpse something of the intricate hierarchy of this church, and of its size and power.

There was no discreet passing of the offering plate here. The audience was told precisely what to give: most of us were to donate ten dollars; pastors and missionaries were to give more. Ushers directed us, one segment of the room at a time, to the platform, where we tossed bills onto a table in front of the vigilant eyes of several preachers.

Perhaps I had hoped for a sign. If so, it had not come. I had found the service joyous and exhilarating, been moved by the piety in the room. I had always believed that the godhead— whether conceived of as an infinite source of love and creativity, the world mind or some ultimate truth—was to be found in all the world's great religions, that mystics in all churches—Jewish, Christian, Buddhist, Hindu, Islamic—arrived at the same insights. It was as if there were a great and universal truth, like a crystal that had been shattered, and each shard retained the full spectrum of the rainbow.

Melanie slept in the back seat as Ginny drove us home. "I've been wanting to go to a national meeting," Ginny said. "They had one in Memphis. All the hotels had signs that said, 'Welcome, Children of God,' and it was so crowded regular travelers couldn't even find rooms. There were white people and Mexican people there, too. And a lot of people from Japan."

Connie and Vivian were talking quietly. "Hey," Ginny said mischievously, "I wonder what happened to that bug." Instantly, Connie pulled up her legs and shrieked.

Ginny pulled into our driveway, and I got out of the car. She got out, too, slipped her arm around my waist and walked me slowly to the house.

QuaLife had set up a Boulder branch, and I found the meetings a reliable source of comfort and strength. I asked Bill to attend some sessions with me. "These people are beginning to mean a lot to me," I said. "I'd really like you to meet them."

"I'm sorry," he responded. "You know I'll always be available when you need me. But the support group is your thing. I'm not comfortable with the idea of sitting around with a bunch of strangers, talking about how I feel." That seemed fair enough.

For me, however, it was continually astonishing and nourishing to hear people I hardly knew talking with no coyness or pretension about the deepest aspects of their lives. It's as if, having been diagnosed with cancer, they had simply decided there was no more time for bullshit.

"I don't mind the way I used to when someone cuts in front of me in traffic," said a man who leaned heavily on a three-pronged cane. He'd already told us that five years ago his doctor had given him a year to live, and that his bones were now deteriorating rather rapidly. "I just think, 'Well, you're in a bigger hurry than me.'

"I've had the most wonderful five years of my life. Me and the wife—we don't postpone the things we want to do anymore. We visit our children. We travel. I've never been happier."

A round little woman talked about her mother's death. "She didn't want to be buried in anything formal, and she had this pretty, lacy nightdress she wanted to be buried in. So that's what I did. One of my friends looked in the casket and said, 'I can't believe you really did it.'

"She sang in a choir and at the funeral all her friends came and sang for her. It was a very joyous thing."

"I think it's beautiful that it was so peaceful for you," said another woman. "I think about if I have to die that I want to die well. I want to find a way to die that means my children can go on with their lives and not be traumatized."

There was one discordant thing about these meetings. At the beginning of each session, each participant in turn rose and explained his or her reason for coming. Some of these people were not cancer patients. I respected those who came to support a sick family member and the therapists whose interest was professional. I even respected those drawn to us by their fear of our disease. But I resented the people who seemed to be there out of curiosity or some strange psychological need I couldn't fathom.

"I just love being with you people," said one such woman. "You're all so wonderful."

"My God," I whispered to Molly, who was sitting next to me. "There are cancer groupies."

"Yes," she said, "and death groupies, too."

If I sometimes had to cope with a frisson of resentment that people who had never had cancer were cluttering up our meetings, I found out later, visiting a different support group, that sometimes people with advanced cancer resented the presence of people like me. They wanted to speak freely and not to hold back for fear of frightening us. They knew, because they had done it, that a cancer patient erects the same kind of barrier between herself and someone with metastasis that most of the world erects between itself and her.

"You are completely other," the world tells us. "I have undertaken a regimen, a way of life, a stance, a kind of thinking that protects me from ever becoming you." And so we say, internally, to those worse off than we: "I had a less aggressive kind of tumor; I had no lymph node involvement; I chose a wiser course of treatment; I am following a more stringent diet—my case is sufficiently different from yours to assure that I will never, never be in your position."

These people look at us silently. They know the difference between us and them. They know that they, too, constructed a list of reasons to expect to stay well forever. But then one day, feeling strong and secure, they'd felt a lump or a small ache. Or received notice from their doctors that the latest blood test revealed tumor activity. Suddenly they had tumbled from the little perch of safety we all cling to into the abyss. It can happen as abruptly to any one of us—or to someone who has never had cancer at all. These dying men and women want to protect us from that knowledge. And they also want to rub our noses in it. But primarily, they want us out of their workshops and sessions so they can talk together without worrying about our feelings at all.

At most community meetings, however, as strong as the desire to make separations was the deep understanding of our common predicament. At one meeting I heard a woman with metastatic ovarian cancer and a very poor prognosis giving careful tips on vitamins and diet to someone who had attended the session only because of a mildly suspicious pap smear.

One night, a couple, Doug and Lois Cox, described Doug's struggle with a cancer that had begun under his tongue and moved to the lymph nodes in his throat. Doug had received a copy of Dr. Bernie Siegel's *Love, Medicine and Miracles* and been impressed by the doctor's approach and by his assertion that patients could exert some control over their physical functions by visualizing and by maintaining a positive state of mind. When Doug was scheduled to have radioactive pins placed in his throat for thirty-six hours, he decided to visualize the blood flowing away from the incisions, and he instructed Lois to direct the blood away, too, speaking aloud to him when he became groggy.

When the doctor came to remove the pins, however, Doug and Lois weren't thinking about blood flow. "Hey," commented the doctor. "This is odd. You're bleeding more now that I'm taking these out than you did when I was putting them in."

Doug used the same techniques to help himself through surgery and chemotherapy. In visualization sessions, he imagined a beaver nibbling away busily on his tumor cells.

Lois began describing how Bernie Siegel had come to give a speech in Denver while Doug was still in treatment. Unable to attend, Doug had sent the doctor a note.

"On Sunday, the phone rang," Lois said. "It was Dr. Siegel. He wanted to speak to Doug, wanted to know how he was doing."

"We talked for a while," said Doug. "You know, I've heard some people think he's a phony, or he's getting kind of tired out and less giving, and I wish I could tell them all about that phone call and what it did for me."

Watching the gratitude and wonder on Doug's and Lois's faces, I once again cursed my own skepticism, wished I could believe as fervently in New Age theory as they did.

Now they were talking about a turning point in Doug's illness.

"We were in the kitchen," said Lois. "I was just fixing dinner, and Doug was feeling really ill. And ..." She turned to him. "Perhaps you should tell this?"

"No," he said. "Go ahead."

"Well, I was just putting the pans on the stove, and—I think we were having chicken—and—Doug was sitting at the table— and I said something—I said ..." Her voice faltered.

"You said I should go ahead and die if I wanted to. You said it was OK to die."

There was pure love in his voice.

"That did it," he said. "I don't really know how. It took the burden off somehow, and I was able to get better."

Sara Wolfe was sitting next to me. Beautiful Sara, who had survived her supposedly incurable cancer by five years, was pregnant. Later in the evening, I asked if I might feel her stomach, and, without a second's self-consciousness, she took my hand and held it firmly against her hard, round belly.

"Wait," she said. "The baby was kicking just a minute ago. Oh, there it is."

Against my palm, the faraway flutter of life.

19
THE SHAMBLING FAMILIAR

Molly slipped quietly into a circle of participants at a QuaLife session. "Hey," I whispered, "it's been a while. How're you doing?"

"I had a metastasis," she said. "But I'm OK."

I didn't know how to respond. She couldn't be OK. A breast cancer metastasis was considered terminal. But she was cheerful and composed. Perhaps I hadn't heard her correctly. I let her comment pass.

A few days later, we met for breakfast at a bustling health food restaurant, where, as she said, "We can be properly virtuous." We ordered scrambled tofu with vegetables and mushrooms. I studied her narrow, smiling face closely, looking for signs of ill health. Were her bones more prominent, her skin tones more yellow? But she looked as trim, neatly dressed and energetic as ever.

A few months earlier, Molly had felt a slight pain along her breastbone, so slight it was barely above the threshold of perception. She went to John Fleagle for a bone scan, "and I did a lot of thinking about the power of words, because when I was going in to see him to get the verdict, I remember writing in my journal, 'I'm going to find out today whether I have cancer or not'—and I thought I did—but isn't it weird, because knowing that will change my life, but I'll be the same. If I've got it, it's been growing for a long time. Today isn't going to change anything. And yet in other ways, today will change everything."

Nothing showed up on the first bone scan, but eventually blood tests indicated that the cancer had returned. "Boy, was that hard," Molly said. "I mean, I really thought I was cured. I was going on three years, and so my hope had grown back. When I originally was diagnosed, I was not willing to convince myself

247

that I was going to be cured because I didn't want to go through the pain of learning that I hadn't been. But then, you know, you keep going back to the doctor and everything's fine and everything's fine and everything's fine, and so you start saying, 'Hey, I think I'm going to make it.' And then you get the diagnosis that says you didn't."

I smothered the fierce little flame of fear that shot up in my chest. I wanted to be calm and helpful for Molly.

She had had to fight feelings of guilt, fear that her own deficiencies had caused the recurrence. "It was one thing if this disease was going to kill me," she said, "but I needed to know in my heart that it wasn't because I hadn't done things right. It wasn't because I hadn't gotten my stress under control or changed my life. ... And I really think that's the two-edged sword of all those self-help books. People who get cured convince themselves that it's all the things they did. But if it is, what about those of us who don't get cured?"

Molly rode across mountains on her bicycle. She hiked miles. She was happily married and the calm, competent administrator of a nonprofit organization. It was hard to imagine anyone whose daily life was more satisfying.

The recurrence brought fear as well as guilt. Molly cried a lot. She went to a therapist. With him she did an exercise in which she pictured her cancer. It looked like a brain, she said, "all alive and glisteny on the outside. And I made a little hole, and I went inside it. It was hollow and dry, like a cave. I used to do a lot of caving when I was younger.

"I found a room that was lit with candles. It had crystals on the wall, and the crystals formed a star, like a Star of David. And there were canisters that had things in them that when you shook them sounded like marbles. So the upshot of all this—I mean, my images are not very sophisticated; they're easy to get to—I now take vitamins—you know, the marbles. And I've developed a really strong spiritual interest."

Molly had begun meditating. She had grown up Catholic, she said, and had fought hard to leave the religion. But recently she had attended some meditation classes given by a monk in Snowmass. "He calls it centering prayer, but he's teaching exactly the same thing that the Buddhists are teaching. All these major religions are teaching the same thing."

Like almost all the cancer patients I'd met, she had become more concerned about other people, less interested in money or status. She had married only a few years earlier, in her forties. She and her husband felt a little cheated, she said, because they would not have much time together. "But it's not in that sort of tragic mode. I've climbed mountains. I've done all kinds of wonderful, exciting things with my life.

"One of the things I've thought about these last months is the idea of what would you do if your world were to end tomorrow? Because that's what you're talking about when you talk about having cancer and dying. Your world's going to end. So what would we do if we all knew that? Well, we'd probably still eat breakfast, and we'd probably still go to the bathroom. You'd have to cook supper, because everybody still would be hungry. It's bad enough to have this stuff; there's no point letting it ruin the joys of today. Today is so precious."

We paid for our meal, hugged each other and promised to meet again soon.

Almost every week, on my video terminal at the paper, I read about experiments that offered hopeful new possibilities for cancer patients. Experiments involving interferon and interleukin, monoclonal antibodies. I learned that eventually doctors would set loose genetically engineered cells that could home in on tumors as swift and clean as a fish darting at a fly. Destroy them. Engulf them. Or simply teach the chaotically replicating cancer cells some sense of order. Surgery, radiation, chemotherapy—the treatments Molly and I had endured—would someday be as out of date as the universal tonsillectomy. But all the articles ended with the same caveat. Patients should not put their hopes in these remedies. It would be years before they were in general use.

It seemed as if Molly were in a small room, in which the walls and ceiling were continuously contracting, and where a couple of high, slotted windows offered the only hope of escape. One window was a bone marrow transplant: a hideous, soul-destroying procedure that offered a 10 percent chance of actually killing her, against a 15 to 30 percent chance of cure. That was an option if the doctor running the experimental program decided she qualified for it. And if her insurance company was willing to pay costs of between one and two hundred thousand dollars.

A second window: she could explore alternative therapies available in Texas, Bermuda, New York State, San Diego, therapies involving enzymes, vitamins, rigid diets and coffee enemas. Some of them seemed to offer some success rate. But since statistics on these regimes were sparse and mutually contra-dictory, choosing one of them would be an act of faith. You'd be tormented continually with the thought that perhaps you'd picked the wrong one.

The final possibility was to accept impending death, seek her doctor's help in alleviating symptoms as they arose and enjoy the precious, dwindling time left to her.

Some time later, I was on a routine visit to Dr. Fleagle. The examination was over, and we were chatting. He told me that I was fine and he expected me to do well, and I began talking about the future of cancer diagnosis and treatment—more in the mode, at that moment, of a journalist than a patient.

"It seems to me there are some ethical dilemmas coming up," I said, "as the ability to predict outstrips the ability to treat. Gene research means they'll be able to tell who's likely to get certain kinds of cancers, but they still won't have cures for them. All they can do is tell cancer-prone people to exert a lot of vigilance.

"I hear that for people who have tumors, they're better able now to analyze them and predict which ones will recur. Since treatment methods haven't kept up with the ability to predict, this doesn't seem like very useful information. I wouldn't want to know the results of a test like flow cytometry, for instance—and I don't know if you did that on my tumor—if there was nothing I could do about a bad result. ..."

"Yes," said Dr. Fleagle, "we did perform flow cytometry."

Again the heavy weight crushing my chest. Again the terrible clarity of the moment, the sense that time had stopped.

"Do you want to know what we found?"

I nodded. He began riffling through the pages of my chart.

"Here it is. Your tumor was aneuploid. That means the tumor cells had an abnormal amount of DNA in them. We couldn't read the S-curve, which measures the rate at which they're dividing."

"That's not good?" I said stupidly.

"Let me explain." He spoke carefully and thoughtfully for several minutes, even drew a diagram for me, but I couldn't absorb what he was saying. I was thinking of what John Day had said a few months earlier: "You had a freaky, aggressive tumor."

At times like this I realized that what I'd learned from the road I'd traveled, any wisdom or resignation or understanding I'd acquired, my proud ability to lead a normal life in the face of cancer—all these things were only a thin skin. The place of fear into which I tumbled at Dr. Fleagle's words, the yawning chasm that opened within me, was always there. It was just that I usually kept it covered, somehow. I thought of a soldier walking along a green jungle path in Vietnam, and how it caved suddenly under his feet, hurling him onto the sharp stakes hidden in the pit beneath.

For three days I fought to regain my equilibrium. "We could have guessed that your tumor would be aneuploid from the fact that it had spread to the lymph nodes," Dr. Fleagle had said. "It doesn't really change anything. The figures I gave you for long-term survival are still the same. Really, all the flow cytometry predicted is that it would have spread to the nodes, and, hey," he smiled sympathetically, "you got to freak out about that months ago. No need to do it again."

I called Doris Olsen and a new friend who had had two mastectomies, Pat Wagenhals. Neither of them knew anything about flow cytometry. Then I tried the National Cancer Institute's hotline and the American Cancer Society, and both organizations sent me studies. While the studies did indicate, in a general way, that an aneuploid tumor meant a worse prognosis, none of them really related very specifically to my case. I realized this method of analyzing tumors simply hadn't been around long enough for a detailed body of research to have arisen around it. Most of what I read bore out Dr. Fleagle's assertion: aneuploidy and a fast S-curve predicted a more aggressive tumor; such a tumor was more likely to have spread to the lymph nodes; I already knew the figures indicating that lymph node involvement meant a poorer prognosis. It was not, however, an automatic death sentence.

I remembered Dr. Wood's suggestion on how to get through the times when the terror became overwhelming. "I'm alive right now," I'd repeat like a mantra. "I'm walking down this street and the clouds are sailing through the sky and I don't know what's going to happen tomorrow, but I'm alive right this minute."

Sometimes I'd go back to the way I'd thought as a child. I was convinced then that the entire world would be incinerated by bombs before I got to grow up. As I drifted into sleep I'd tell myself, even if there is going to be a war, it won't be tonight. So I'll still be able to eat a fried egg with toast and butter for breakfast. And I'll still be able to go over to my friend Sheila's and play this weekend, because there won't be a war before then. ...

Eventually, the knowledge that I had had an aggressive tumor became simply one more piece of information, dropped from the panicky forefront of my imagination to a low-level but persistent concern.

For the next few weeks, however, the sharpened stakes lay in wait for me. Joe Devon, a co-worker, left for a week to visit his dying mother in another state. When he returned, he told me in detail how awful his experience had been. His mother had seen him come in and had attempted to raise herself from the bed, but all she could do was whisper his name, her arms uselessly extended toward him, and fall back on the bed. He had never understood before, Joe said, just how very terrible it was to die of cancer.

His mother had had breast cancer nine years earlier. She had appeared to recover completely. But routine hip surgery had revealed breast cancer cells in her bones.

"Oh, boy," Joe said suddenly. "I shouldn't have told you any of this."

I said, "It's OK. You had to."

I had been working with an intern, a tall, dark young man who was a very dedicated and talented photographer. One afternoon he brought in a book called *Exploding into Life*. It was an account of her breast cancer experience by Dorothea Lynch. Photographs by her companion, the brilliant photographer Eugene Richards, accompanied the text.

"I thought you'd like to read this," said the intern. "The way she writes kind of reminds me of the way you do. She even writes about her garden like you do."

The book sat unopened on my desk for a few days. One evening, just as I was about to leave work, I began paging through it. I read how Dorothea Lynch had discovered her cancer—how it felt small and hard like the cap of a tube of toothpaste. I saw Richards's stark photograph of her bloody, fresh mastectomy. The intern was right: I loved Lynch's prose style, her honesty and imagination—and the prose was matched by the intensity and power of the photographs.

Lynch was a poet who worked as a journalist. I felt a strong sense of kinship. I would write to this woman; I would tell her what her book meant to me.

Now she was writing about a recurrence, saying something about how the doctors would probably pull her through, as they had before. I turned to the end of the book. There was a note by Eugene Richards. "For almost two years I have been sleeping half on the floor or against the wall, not wanting to move Dorothea's notebooks and diaries off my bed. On hot, humid nights, pages, loose from their binding, stick to my back and my shoulders; in winter, when I try to turn over, they crackle like dried leaves. Still, I can't move them. Almost everything else that belonged to her— clothes, car, jewelry—has been donated to charity, sold, or carried off by friends. ..."

I had to read this quiet postscript twice before I would let myself understand.

Dorothea Lynch was dead. I began to cry. I had known her an hour, and she was dead, this friend, this fellow sufferer, this sister. Weeping in the deserted office, I didn't know anymore who I was crying for—Dorothea Lynch, Joe's mother, Molly, myself, all of us. It was some time before I could put on my coat and leave for home.

The Sunday Magazine Editors' Conference was scheduled for Dallas in April. This was the same conference I had planned to attend a year earlier, when I had found the lump in my breast and called Caryn, telling her I was too frightened to leave home, too frightened to fly. It seemed very important that I go this year.

I was a little intimidated about being away from Bill and Anna, but the editors turned out to be a jokey, intelligent lot; the hotel where we stayed was sumptuous; I found I was enjoying myself. Halfway through the first day of presentations, business discussion and panels, I found myself sitting next to the magazine editor for a very fine East Coast newspaper. He started when he heard my name, then asked if I had written a story about breast cancer that had appeared in the *Boulder Daily Camera*. It seemed his wife, too, had the disease. Soon, we were ensconced in a quiet corner of the lobby, talking.

His wife was fighting a recurrence, and he was angry about the way cancer was covered in the media, the endless stories about plucky little kids who beat the disease.

"It's as if they were saying that the ones who don't survive aren't courageous or don't have the same passion for life," he said. "Brave, strong people sometimes die."

"And horrible, whiny people sometimes survive," I said. "You know, my analyst says that healing doesn't always mean getting better. Sometimes it means dying well."

The editor's face lit up. "That's great." He thought a moment. "What does it mean?"

We talked on. He told me that he and his wife had two small children, and that when she was first diagnosed, she had turned away from them, appearing to reject them. I thought about Karen DuBose and her futile, desperate attempt to spare her children the pain of loving her.

The editor also explained how hard it was for him to deal with his feelings. He didn't want to discuss them with his wife; he thought it would be wrong to add his anxiety and fear to the burden she was carrying.

Later, in my room, I thought about Bill and the optimistic, stoical demeanor he had maintained almost without a break since my diagnosis. He had been quite willing to talk about the structure of our lives, to plan for a more aware and integrated future for the family, but he said nothing about any sorrow or fear he might be feeling. Periodically, one of our friends—Lynn or Louise—would ask if he wanted to talk. Or Gunner would invite him for beers and a little man-to-man talk. But Bill insisted, cheerfully and steadily, that he was fine, that he didn't need help. Pondering all this as I sank into sleep in Dallas, I resolved to press him more strongly on my return home.

The conference ended on Saturday noon, but several of us were staying the night in Dallas in order to take advantage of cheaper weekend travel rates. The editor of a San Francisco magazine and a woman who edited a magazine in Oregon suggested that the three of us go out to dinner.

We found a seat by the window at a trendy restaurant with a candy-slick, brightly colored decor and huge, crimson-backed menus. You could order an elaborate meal composed of eight or more courses, or a truncated, four-course version. I ordered the latter, knowing that the *Camera* would question a large bill. Mark and Marilyn decided to sample everything.

Course after course arrived at the table, many of them no more than a tiny nibble of something savory, garnished in contrasting colors and set dead center on a huge, geometrically patterned, blue and white plate.

We ate, tasted each other's dishes and talked. Mark told us about the ridiculous cost of housing in the Bay Area; we discussed the difficulties of finding good freelancers; the overall direction being taken by our newspapers.

Eventually, Mark stood up and went outside to smoke a cigarette. Marilyn began telling me about a woman she worked with who had just received a diagnosis of breast cancer. It made her feel awkward, Marilyn said. She didn't quite know how to handle it.

I thought I could help. "I've had breast cancer," I said. "I've been in treatment all year and have just finished."

She was not particularly interested. We exchanged a couple of sentences, and Mark came back to the table. He hadn't heard me say that I'd had cancer, but he did catch the tail-end of our discussion.

"My mother-in-law had breast cancer," he said. "Terrible thing. She had a lumpectomy and radiation and they thought she was fine, but two years later, it came back and killed her."

Smoke drifted toward us from a neighboring table. I knew cigarette smoke was a strong tumor promoter. I turned my head to try and avoid inhaling, but the smoke slithered down my throat. I tasted ashes.

Marilyn leaned forward eagerly. "Oh, I know," she said. "It is a terrible thing. The most terrible thing there is. My father died of cancer. He just wasted away until he was all bones."

I looked at her, mutely pleading, hoping she'd remember my plight and stop.

"At the end they had him hooked up to a continuous morphine drip," she said. "It wasn't enough to stop the pain. He kept moaning and crying, begging for more painkiller."

I was trying to hold my breath, trying not to listen and to let her words become a meaningless blur of sound, but smoke was dribbling steadily into my lungs.

"Even after he died, I couldn't get the way he looked at the end out of my mind. I still can't. When I see old people on the street and they look wasted, the skin hanging on their bones the way his did ... I just can't bear it."

My chest ached. The restaurant was hot and noisy. Periodically a word surfaced from the flood of Marilyn's talk: "agony," "emaciated," "screaming."

I excused myself from the table and pushed my way into the bathroom. There I closed myself in a cubicle and leaned against the wall, struggling for breath, yearning for the sight of my daughter and the comfort of Bill's arms.

A few days later I was safely home. "Do you remember that first evening, when I'd seen Dr. Day and he'd told me I probably had cancer?" I asked Anna one morning.

"Yes," she said. "Daddy and I went out on the porch, and I asked him what would happen if you died. He said we'd be very sad, and on some level we'd never get over it, but eventually we'd get on with our lives because Mommy wouldn't want us to be miserable forever."

I thought about how I'd urged Bill to remarry if I died. I was greedy for my family now. I wanted to clutch my world and never let it go. I said, "Like hell I wouldn't."

Anna looked at me, startled, and we both collapsed in laughter.

Later, I was sitting with Bill on the porch. The apple tree was resplendent with blossom, holding its branches low and wide like a peacock displaying his tail. Petra and McDuff lay close at hand, McDuff jealously guarding a much-gnawed stick.

I told Bill about the editor I'd talked to in the lobby, his inability to express his vulnerabilities to his cancer-stricken wife. Did Bill have the same problem, I wanted to know. How had he felt in those early days?

"It was like the Alice in Wonderland thing," he said. "All of a sudden we took a pill and we were in a whole new reality. The house was the same; the dogs were the same; the trees were the same; everything was the same—except you were different. And we were all different because of what it could mean."

It was as if he'd suddenly found himself underwater, Bill said. "You have a certain amount of breath and you can either panic or you can see the other side and say, well, to get from here to there is going to take a lot of breath control. And you start swimming like hell, and you have to let go of little bits of air as you go. You have to be very disciplined or you're not going to make it to the other side."

"Do you remember when I crawled in bed and you pulled the covers off and yelled at me not to lie there and let myself die?" I asked.

257

"I had this superstitious thing that if you gave up you would die. And it smacked of loss of control, which I don't like." He laughed. "Hey, it's not manly. Besides, you British are supposed to know how to keep a stiff upper lip."

"Did you think about how you'd feel if I died?"

"That's real hard to talk about. You and I have gotten so into each other's skin and blood and aura and energy over the years. On one level, it'd be like any other day. Because a lot of times we just go off and do our own thing. Life would go on just like life goes on. Except there would be this tremendous empty hollow place. The predominant feeling would be one of real loss and real sadness because I wouldn't be able to argue with you and kick you in the ass and tickle you, get in fights with you, go for long walks. ... It would be like getting an arm or a leg chopped off. You'd learn to get around and to do things, and there'd be this big chunk of you that just wouldn't be there." He paused. "So you're not allowed to die."

Bill himself had been changing his life, quietly and steadily, ever since the putative heart attack eight years earlier. His decision to leave his job and become an independent consultant had been part of this. In the last few weeks, with his encouragement and support, I had finally decided to give up my job as a department head at the *Daily Camera* and to ask for a part-time writing position. This would strain our finances, but it would at least enable me to keep some steady income, as well as my health insurance.

"It's ironic," Bill said, "but in many ways this has been the happiest year of my life. I've loved working here at home. You and I have spent much more time together, and also with Anna. I think she appreciates it. At any rate, she's really blossoming.

"And you're putting up with less bullshit in everything. You've decided you're not going to do work that isn't satisfying to you. You're writing. You're doing your creative work. You said, 'I'm not going after the big prizes in the business world; I'm not going to be a manager.' All the ego things we spend so much of our time on just dropped away. What was left was the real kernel of what you wanted your life to be."

20
THE GIFT

Her name was Luanne Hyman, and she lay naked on the table under huge, round lights, her arms spread as if she were being crucified, her wrists Velcro'd to supporting bars. Her eyes were taped shut, and a tube going into her throat was secured with tape that obscured the lower half of her face. Her breasts were bruised green, yellow and blue from her biopsies, and lines had been drawn on them with purple marker. A nurse, Marianna Lewis, washed her abdomen down with Betadine soap, applied with a square sponge on a stick. The color was a kind of iodine rust, deepening to blood.

"It's a challenge to wash the skin without taking off all the marks," Marianna said.

A couple of weeks earlier, Dr. Day had suggested that perhaps I should watch him in surgery. "It might help your healing process to know exactly what it is," he'd said. "Round off some of the corners for you."

"If it isn't too scary," I'd said, "I'd like to watch a mastectomy, even though I didn't have one. And perhaps I could interview you. Sort of get an idea of what this world of cancer looks like from your perspective."

The interview completed, I'd dithered for some time about watching surgery, unsure whether I would become more or less afraid of it, more or less accepting of the surgery that I had undergone. I called Antonio Wood. He said that since this was one of my worst fears, it would be good to face it. I talked to Darrell Sifford, a columnist for the *Philadelphia Inquirer* who had written about watching a heart surgery similar to the one he'd had himself.

"I'd encourage you to do it," he said. "It gives you a sense of how skilled and controlled the work is. It made me feel much more confidence in the care I'd received."

But Ed Bryant, master of horror fiction, described how he'd once planned to witness an operation on a dog and had fainted watching the vet prepare to make the first cut.

Now, for better or for worse, I was standing in the operating room, three or four feet away from Luanne, masked, gowned, capped and with paper boots on my feet.

Marianna and another nurse began draping Luanne's body with blue cloth, leaving only a square of skin around her breast exposed.

"She has multifocal intraductal carcinoma of the right breast," John Day explained to me. "In situ. Most breast cancers arise from the duct system, some from the lobules. Hers has not spread out of the duct."

John preferred to perform lumpectomies whenever possible, but in Luanne's case, the cancer had originated in more than one site, making mastectomy imperative. Because no cancer cells had invaded beyond the duct, however, her prognosis was excellent. A biopsy on the left breast had shown "mild intraductal hyperplasia," John said. "We'll follow it like a hawk."

Reconstruction was to begin on the right breast immediately after the mastectomy, and the left breast, too, would be lifted a little, so that they were symmetrical.

John nodded toward the unconscious form on the table. "She doesn't have any qualms," he said approvingly, standing up to walk out of the room. "She just moves along with things."

I knew this was true. I had interviewed Luanne the day before, and she had talked about her faith that everything would be all right and her trust in and affection for John Day. Just before her second biopsy, she said, her husband had told Day it was her birthday: "They sent me in, and Dr. Day started working. Then he stopped, walked around the back of the table and put those huge hands on the sides of my face. And he said, 'Why didn't you tell me it was your birthday? We could have done this tomorrow.' I said, 'I didn't want to wait till tomorrow, sir.'

"So he and those two nurses stood there on the other side of the table, giggling and singing happy birthday. They were so silly."

During the interview, and on the morning before surgery, Luanne had been calm and cheerful. "I had my falling apart, screaming, crying fit Wednesday. I was talking to my husband on the phone, and I just came apart at the seams. He came home, and I was busy vacuuming the floor and crying.

"I spent about half an hour saying everything that came to my mind. 'I don't want to die.' 'I can't have cancer.' 'What are we going to do?' 'How can I afford to be off work?' and got it all out of my system.

"Surgery doesn't frighten me, and cancer doesn't frighten me. Whatever comes along comes along. God never asked me to take on anything that I couldn't handle."

Luanne's chest rose and fell slowly under the blue cloths. I remembered the surprise she'd planned for her husband. "I went shopping with my best friend last weekend, and I passed the chocolate shop, and I couldn't resist," she'd said the night before. "I have this little box with a pair of truffles in it, and they look like a nice set of matched breasts. So we're going to sneak them in when they bring me to surgery. I got a very sweet card. After all he's been through, he deserves it. My mom's going to give him the card and the truffles. On the inside of the lid I wrote, 'Promise of things to come.'"

The plastic surgeon, Dr. Scott Replogle, came in, wiping his hands. Behind him came John Day. Both men were wearing rubber gloves. John had green clogs on his feet. (I thought this an amusing eccentricity but learned later that they were nonslip and good for his posture at the table.) There was a double strand of meditation beads around his neck. Strapped to Replogle's forehead was what looked like a miner's lamp.

The doctors consulted briefly over Luanne's still body. The table was adjusted. Replogle, considerably shorter than the lanky Day, positioned himself on a low step. Day began cutting. I couldn't really see this: Replogle's back and both surgeons' hands obscured my line of vision. I noticed a faint smell of burning.

"This instrument can both cut and cauterize," said Replogle, "depending on the button pressed by the surgeon."

"It's a major advance in surgery," Day said. "We used to put a clamp on each vessel and tie it off. It took six hours to do a mastectomy. This came out in the seventies."

"Is it like laser surgery?"

"Laser is a high-tech way of doing the same thing; it's a more precise delivery of the energy. Clinically, it doesn't make much difference. Electrocautery is just as good and less expensive. Laser is useful for the back of the eye, places in the throat, hard-to-get-at surgery."

The burning smell became intense. The room was very cold. One of the nurses slipped me a step like the one Replogle was standing on. Once on it, I saw that an elliptical opening had been created clear across Luanne's breast, and Replogle was holding up the skin so that John could carefully cut away the flesh. There was a moment of sheer horror—the gaping red-rimmed wound, the yellow fat, singed black in places.

The atmosphere in the room was quiet, concentrated. Simon and Garfunkel played softly in the background; Marianna kept a watchful eye on Luanne.

I had thought of surgery as an atavistic, dark and bloody event. Now I saw that it was something else. I remembered John Day talking to me about the church he'd attended as a small boy in Montgomery, Alabama, and how he'd become transfixed by a stained-glass window showing a sick man being healed by Christ.

"I would always just sit there and gaze at it while these boring lectures and sermons were going on, and all this ritual was going on—sitting up, kneeling down, standing up and singing hymns. ..."

Later he said, "I think there is a kind of natural predisposition that makes us all choose what we wish to do with ourselves, makes us choose how we wish to spend our time in life. ... I guess I have to say that it's a matter of divine providence that these kinds of decisions are made for you. You are led into those decisions, and you are given the gift that is necessary for you to stand by someone's side and open their body and go in there and do what has to be done."

"It's astonishing," I whispered to Marianna. "This is the one thing everyone I know is most afraid of. But for you guys it's just a day's work. I walk into the newspaper office and turn on my computer; John comes in here and cuts someone open."

Behind Luanne's head, the anesthesiologist, Dr. Dick Balkins, sat by a bank of instruments, unmoving, watching them closely. He pointed to a column on the bank. "This tells me, with each breath, how much the volume is. This," pointing to another, "tells me how much carbon dioxide is in her bloodstream. Our normal breathing is geared by the amount of carbon dioxide we need to get rid of, not the amount of oxygen we need to take in. This equipment lets me keep her at a physiological level that's normal or a little below normal. There's a pulse oxymeter—a clip on her finger. It tells me how much oxygen is in her bloodstream."

In a Plexiglass cylinder, a kind of bellows rose and fell. Green numbers glinted on the machine bank.

"You really take over a person's functions and keep them going," said Dr. Balkins.

"So you're her guardian angel," I said.

"I've never been called that before, but, yeah, that describes it."

He went on, "It used to be that all you had was a stethoscope. I started in 1950. Between then and 1965, you had an airpiece and a blood pressure pump you pumped up with your hand.

"We used a dozen different things for her," he nodded toward Luanne. "A combination of drugs to put her to sleep. She'll be awake five minutes after John's done. We keep people in a light plane of anesthesia so that they wake up quickly, without problems."

"All right," John said, working on the exposed breast. "Here's an ivory quiz. How many animals can you name that have ivory?" His tone was jocular, erudite. He sounded like a popular professor quizzing a class.

"Elephants," said one of the nurses.

"Elk. Whales," said Marianna.

"What kind of whales?"

"Killer whales. Sperm whales."

Replogle's hand followed Day's, pressing a white cloth against the wound.

Day carefully fingered the flesh out. "What other animals?" Silence. "What about a walrus?"

"A walrus has ivory?" said Replogle.

"Yes, sir. And you don't have to kill any to get it."

Luanne's nipple stood exposed on a kind of stem of flesh. Then the entire mass toppled slowly and forlornly to one side. I turned away and sat down. Marianna had given me a stool earlier, whispering, "Put your head down if you feel dizzy."

She had also told me that this was not a painful surgery for the patient, because the surgeon did not cut through muscle as in the old Halsted radical. In addition, some nerves were severed during the node dissection. This minimized pain, though, as I knew from my own experience, it meant a permanent numbness in some places under the arm.

The muscle along Luanne's chest wall, exposed, glistened red. John told me he was using the same incision to cut out the lymph nodes, but all I saw was a jumble of hands and instruments. Once or twice, Luanne's abdomen heaved as if she were sighing deeply.

John placed the nodes in a steel pan, cut part of the flesh away from them. I was reminded of a housewife cleaning off a piece of liver. The tissue went to the lab for analysis, Marianna told me later, and the waste was incinerated.

Marianna carried away a jar. I could see the nipple through the transparent side.

When she returned, John said quietly to her, "The family would like to know that the breast tissue has been removed and that reconstruction is proceeding on the right, and that she is doing well." Marianna nodded and left the room.

John was talking about another patient. "I met her mammogram before I met her. The radiologist wasn't sure she had cancer. But I could see there was a densification, a subtle architectural disturbance. We're doing surgery, but there's a problem with chemotherapy. Her daughter is against it. She's very holistic, but she's ignorantly holistic."

He slid in the drain. If I'd realized how far in it went, I thought, I'd have worried less about mine coming out by accident.

Dr. Replogle put a round, textured expander into the cavity on Luanne's chest. "This locks into the tissue, and the tissue stretches with it," he said. "It's an empty silicone bag, and you inject saline into it. As she heals, you add more saline until it's the right size. Eventually, I'll take it out and put in a permanent implant. This minimizes stress on the area and modifies the tissue as it heals to allow space for the implant."

The nurses confirmed that all the instruments, needles and sponges had been counted. John began stitching Luanne's breast together over the implant. "The stitches underneath will dissolve," he said. The cut looked so clear-edged and defined that it was hard to imagine the edges growing back together again. But it was a great relief to see the contour of the breast filled out.

John said, "I love scrimshaw. I love marine mammal ivory. But I can't tell you anything about it chemically."

"It would be some variant of enamel, wouldn't it?" said Replogle.

"The market took off because President Kennedy loved scrimshaw," said John, a few seconds later.

"Oh yes, I remember," said the anesthesiologist.

"There are strict laws governing ivory: where you can get it, how you can ship it. There's a big market for mastodons and woolly mammals. You don't have to kill those animals, just dig it up. And the ivory is beautiful. Fossilized."

Replogle worked on Luanne's other breast. He said, "I'm taking a tuck out of the bottom and giving her a bit of a lift. I'll broaden the base when I put the implants in both sides. I'd have had trouble duplicating the size and shape of this breast without modifying it."

This breast was neatly closed, and John began stapling it shut with tiny, gleaming staples, using what looked like a regular staple gun. "It looks painful," he said, seeing me wince, "but these are painless to remove." Later, Luanne confirmed this.

"One of the things I like about surgery," John had said in the interview, "is that it's a definitive statement on a disease process.

You're going to go in there and mechanically correct something that can't be corrected any other way, or you're going to take something out, or in some cases you're going to put something into a body to make it work better.

"To me, surgery seems like a natural thing to do when a body is broken so badly that it needs fast help. When you don't have the healing capacity of a Christ and you can't make a miracle happen instantly, you've got to be able to try and act as an instrument that'll turn it around as quickly as possible. And often medicines are not strong enough.

"And I suppose in the midst of every surgeon's nature is a sort of fire that burns for that kind of action.

"It's a mechanical craft. It satisfies my right brain and my left brain. It keeps the rational, logical, linear, deductive side of me in balance with the artistic, symbolic, philosophical, expressive side. And I get to do that not only in the operating room, but with patients before and after their surgery. And their families, too, if I'm allowed to."

"When we first met," I said, "you seemed a little cold, a little aloof. I felt that if I wasn't brave and cheerful every minute, you would be irritated and turn away from me. And that was terrifying, because you were my doctor and my life was in your hands."

The response was thoughtful. He admitted that for a long time he'd had difficulty dealing with patients who became emotional, particularly women, in part because he hadn't dealt fully with his own fears of his mortality. "But that's changing now," he said. "I think more lately about my own limited time on this earth. I think about my children a lot, and how difficult it would be for them if I weren't around. I can feel that in my patients, and I can feel their life and experiences and all the wonderful things that we get to enjoy as human beings. I can see all that getting snatched away from them, and their anguish and their frustration and their anger.

"Some, however, accept it with total calm resolve and a magnanimity and humility that leave me baffled."

The nurses wound gauze around Luanne's chest, then taped the bandages neatly into place. I wondered if she would be frightened when the time came to take them off. I wanted to tell her how beautifully shaped her breast was, how skilled and precise the work on it had been.

John walked away from the table. While he sat on a stool and wrote his notes, the nurses clustered around Luanne. They freed her wrists from the Velcro, took away the drapes, covered her with a blanket. "You're waking up now," they said. "You're doing fine." The anesthesiologist, holding her head deftly and tenderly in his hands, removed the tube from her throat. She coughed. Her skin was livid. A nurse untaped her eyes. "We have to tape them because sometimes when people are that deeply asleep their eyes roll back and stay open, and they get very dry," Marianna explained.

Dr. Day walked to the table. He touched Luanne's cheek. "Everything went fine," he said. "You got a good result. Everything's going to be all right."

She gave two hideous, loud gasps.

Then she smiled.

21
CODA

The man who came to me in my dream was slender, with a grave demeanor and kind eyes. His dark hair receded a little on his forehead, just as my father's had, and he had my father's enigmatic smile. He stopped inside the garden gate and reached into a burlap bag. "I've brought your order."

He handed me a paper sack containing bulbs. On the front, it said "Magnolias." In the dream I couldn't quite remember what magnolias were, but I had a hazy idea that they were fragrant and very beautiful. Next, he pulled a hard, triangular object from his pocket. It was the size and color of those glossy chestnuts we used to call conkers in England.

"Here," he said. I knew without being told that I had to drop this living thing into water, and then it would soften, divide and grow into something tender and edible.

Finally, the thin man drew forth a clay pot. At first, I saw only that it was filled with earth. Then I looked closer. A sprinkling of the tiniest flowers imaginable covered the soil, as if a warm wind had gently breathed them onto the loamy surface—bluebells, violets, lacy miniature hyacinths.

"That'll be fourteen dollars," said the man. "I'll be bringing more next month."

That's when I understood that his gifts carried a responsibility with them. In my waking life—despite my seed order—I had half decided not to put in a garden. It was clear to me that I needed to spend more time with Bill and Anna, more time on my writing. Besides, there had already been too many summers when I'd planted in spring only to allow the entire plot to be taken over by weeds and insects in the dry heat of midsummer, too many Saturdays of feeling guilty because I wanted to read or walk the dogs instead of hoeing, weeding and mulching. But the dream's message was unequivocal. It was spring. A biological imperative was at work. It was time to turn over the soil.

April always tended to bring such dreams with it: unabashed parables of growth and fertility. I would dream that I had gone out into the winter garden and found it filled with treasures—carrots and lavender, unnameable little golden fruits, things I couldn't remember planting. Frequently eggs and newborn babies entered the swirl of images. This was not subtle stuff.

I got the spade from the shed and went into the garden; since I had neglected fall cleanup, it was in a sorry state. The dried stems of last year's weeds waved forlornly; new weed growth was greening the soil; the rhubarb, ready to push through, was being smothered by a huge mound of autumn leaves. The Christmas tree dropped its needles on the raspberry patch; I had placed it there to help acidify the soil.

I raked the leaves away from the poor, blanched rhubarb stems, breaking some of them in the process. When I nibbled on the end of one, I noticed it was a trifle bitter, less robust in taste than usual. Still, it's hard to deter rhubarb. I was sure the roots would get going again, sending up stalk after sourly tongue-teasing stalk, until Bill and Anna begged for a respite from all the rhubarb fools, crumbles and pies that resulted. Finally, the plants would send up their flowers, holding those bulbous growths that look like truncated cauliflowers aloft as proudly as if they were air-perfuming crimson roses.

I tossed the remnants of the Christmas tree over the fence and began digging. I had never been a very efficient gardener. Because my work at the newspaper demanded clarity and decisiveness, I enjoyed gardening differently: puttering, pawing at things, getting stained with earth and soaked with water, generally messing around. My vegetables never found themselves in straight rows: baby plants meandered and strayed. I would plant a circle of lettuce around a flagstone that just happened to be sitting in a corner, place a lily where a row of spinach had suddenly, inexplicably thinned to nothing. I paid no attention to the fact that it's easier to weed, hoe and mulch if you can go between straight rows.

As a result of these odd planting habits, my hours in the garden were almost as full of surprises as my dreams. On this particular morning, I found a tiny stand of parsley nestled against some sprouting onion tops; a couple of carrots left over from last year's harvest, pushing their energy into fresh, bright green fronds.

As I spaded the remarkably soft and yielding earth, I paused continually to make decisions. There were dozens of clumps of onions. Some I dug up (saving them carefully for the kitchen); some I divided and replanted; some I left in place. The mint was easy. I knew it tended to take over completely, so I could uproot every plant I found, knowing that bouquets of the fragrant leaves were bound to pop up later, and I could decide then to let one mound flourish.

Then there were some vibrant little strawberry plants. I had dug up their patch the previous year because it had yielded very few fruits. But they were so full of life. I just couldn't make up my mind about them. First I'd grit my teeth and spade one up, tossing it aside like a weed. Then I'd dig carefully around another. Finally, I'd rescue one of the orphans I'd uprooted and tenderly replant it.

I knew, of course, that the work would go much faster if I rented a Rototiller, but I couldn't bear the thought of mincing up the myriad earthworms who were going about their job of aerating the soil.

With a weathered wooden stake, I traced a furrow in the earth by the fence. Then I poured some seeds for sugar snap peas onto the palm of my hand and began placing them one by one into the trough. I pushed the earth into place over them, patting and shaping it like a kid playing in sand at the beach. Further into the garden, I did the same for the carrot seeds. It was so hard to imagine a full-blown carrot contained in each of these tiny grains, these fragments of nail parings. Planting them was an act of faith.

My last round of tests—a mammogram and lung X-ray, several blood tests—had revealed nothing threatening, and both Dr. Day and Dr. Fleagle had said they were pleased with my progress and optimistic about my prognosis. I'd be going in for tests every few months and continuing on the Chinese herbs. I leaned on my spade and rested a moment. I thought about how last year's debris—the rotting leaves and stems and fruits—would fertilize the tender shoots of this year's garden. I thought about the blind worms pushing through the clumps of soil and the reaching filaments of root. And I thought about the last year—the odd flashes of pure joy, the constant fear that underlay my daily living and became acute with every freckle, cough, headache or misspoken word. And I thought, I am alive. *Alive.* Can anyone, anywhere, with any assurance, say more?

APPENDIX A
POSTSCRIPT

During the first year after a cancer diagnosis, most of your energy is focused on simply surviving—both emotionally and physically. Once I'd gotten through that year, and this book was completed, I began looking around at the larger picture. It isn't a pleasant one.

In the last year a scandal has arisen that rivals the scandal surrounding the Dalkon Shield. Hundreds of women are claiming injury from the silicone gel implants used in reconstruction after mastectomy. I personally interviewed one young woman who had lost her ability to work, maintain a relationship or live a normal life because of implants. I received a phone message from another who said in a faint voice that she had very little time left and begged for information on any known cure for silicone poisoning. There is none. At present the FDA has restricted the use of these implants, and they are being tested for potential dangers. The response of manufacturers and much of the medical profession to this issue has been eerily reminiscent of the response to the Dalkon Shield controversy in the seventies: obfuscation, avoidance, slick PR kits and out-and-out lies.

The incidence of breast cancer continues to soar, but only a couple of solutions are bruited about in the national discussion on the topic. In the name of prevention, women everywhere are urged to get mammograms and to examine their own breasts. Huge amounts of public money are expended on educational campaigns, and, needless to say, equally huge amounts are taken in by mammogram centers. Now, I believe that an annual mammogram is a good idea for every woman over fifty (the benefits for low-risk women in their forties have yet to be proven). I also think that mammograms should be made available to poor and rural women, and that the accuracy and efficiency of mammogram units should be monitored. These are all good, though limited, actions. But prevention? Once a malignant tumor is found in your breast, you have cancer. You haven't prevented anything. It's true, you're more likely to survive if the tumor is found early, but millions of mammograms, decades of self-examination aren't going to change the basic contour of the problem or the irrefutable fact that more and more of us are getting breast cancer, and we're getting it younger and younger.

Another much publicized approach: In a nationwide trial, healthy women at high risk for breast cancer are being offered the same drug I take daily in the hope of preventing recurrence: tamoxifen. This drug shows great promise in cancer treatment. But it also carries risks. It can cause blood clots and eye problems; it slightly increases the possibility of endometrial cancer. It also causes liver tumors—particularly ugly and aggressive ones—in rats. No one really knows what the effects of long-term ingestion will be in people, as only five thousand women so far have taken tamoxifen for more than five years. For a symptom-free woman to take this unproven drug seems to me the height of foolishness.

One other approach favored by media pundits and some medical personnel is dietary manipulation. They point out that Japanese women have a much lower incidence of breast cancer than do American women, and they become much more susceptible to the disease when they have lived here for some years and switched to the high-fat American diet. *Post hoc ergo propter hoc.* Of course, this way of thinking sets aside the possibility that other variables are at work. Perhaps the air or the water in Japan is different; perhaps people's habits of work or play vary from ours. Perhaps Japanese women don't ingest estrogen. Perhaps they're protected by the soy products in their diet.

A large national experiment set up to explore the correlation between breast cancer and fat consumption found no link. Critics claim that that's because the diet eaten by people on the low-fat arm of the experiment still contained 30 percent fat—too much for the diet to exert any protective effect. These critics also say that the habit of eating a low-fat diet must begin in childhood if it's to avert illness. (Though their childhood diets apparently were of little help to those Japanese women who came to the American diet late in life.)

But there's also the troublesome fact that a link between very low cholesterol and a slightly elevated cancer risk keeps appearing in other experiments.

There's no question that diet plays a role in keeping us healthy. It makes sense to eat a lot of fruits, grains and vegetables, which are known to inhibit the formation of certain cancers, to eat fat only in moderation, to add known anticancer foods and vitamins to your diet, to exercise and otherwise maintain a healthful lifestyle. On the other hand, you probably don't want to hear from me about the joggers, vegetarians and fitness fanatics I've known who got cancer, do you?

Mammograms, tamoxifen, a change in lifestyle, none of these offers any real solution. There are three topics that must be vigorously addressed if we are to deal rationally and compassionately with the problem: root cause, money for research and universal health care.

Root cause. I have seen reams of printed material and listened to hours of testimony, and no one ever asks the simple question: Why is this happening? The possibility that our exposure to estrogen is to blame—in meat, as well as in birth control pills and estrogen replacement therapy—is one hypothesis that must be investigated.

There are others. Thirty years ago, Rachel Carson warned us in her book *Silent Spring* that the chemicals saturating our environment might eventually kill us. We're now facing a massive increase in cancer rates. Could there be a connection? Farmers are more prone than the rest of the population to certain kinds of cancers, and a small, recent study showed that women with breast cancer also had higher concentrations of pesticides in their breast tissue. Now a large study is beginning that may answer some of these questions in ten years' time. Meanwhile, industry and the military continue to spew out pollution. The truth is, we don't

274

have ten years. How many of us have to die before someone decides that chemicals should be banned until proved safe, not poured into air, food, water and soil until proved harmful?

Money for research. The immunological approach to cancer, along with rapidly accelerating research into the human genome, offers a real possibility of cure or at least long-term control of cancer, though this may come ten, twenty or thirty years in the future. When it does, the surgeries, radiation treatments and chemotherapies we currently endure will seem savage and futile. On the threshold of these extraordinary discoveries, it's crucial that the pace of research be maintained.

After a great deal of lobbying by activist groups, $200 million was added to the existing $133 million for breast cancer research in 1992. This is a good beginning, but it's a fraction of what we need. We must make sure that this funding stays in place and continues to grow. And we should insist on patient–doctor supervision of research, so that scientists use the money in the best ways possible, deal compassionately with patients and remain focused on the search for a cure, not on prestige and building wasteful institutional empires.

Thanks to the work of AIDS activists, the release of promising experimental drugs to dying patients has been accelerated. The same courtesy is not currently extended to cancer patients. That has to change.

Universal health care. My friend Molly, like thousands of other cancer patients, was denied by her insurance company the bone marrow transplant that represented the only hope of saving her life.

Every day we read stories about cases like this in the newspaper: patients whose friends and families are holding bake sales and organizing walkathons to pay for needed treatment. These stories are framed as heroic and—it's to be hoped—finally triumphant sagas. Nobody speaks of the utter obscenity of forcing someone who's desperately ill or dying to figure out how much her life is worth. Nobody says it's a sin to make that person spend what may be the last weeks of life suing an insurance company or deciding whether or not to mortgage her family's future, her children's education.

For every brave struggle you read about, there are thousands of quiet deaths.

You rarely hear about the myriad smaller payments routinely refused by insurance companies. I have friends who have gone without diagnostic tests, antinausea drugs, chemotherapies, all requested by doctors, because of the recalcitrance of their insurance companies.

In addition, the various payers—insurance companies, HMOs, Medicare and Medicaid—attempt to contain costs by relentlessly second-guessing doctors, delaying payments or denying them altogether. Dr. Fleagle once explained to me that he spends between 10 and 15 percent of his time dealing with the various insurers.

I know that this kind of pressure, along with the fact that HMOs and PPOs are increasingly dictating patients' choices, forcing some patients to leave physicians they've known for years in favor of doctors picked by the insurer, is driving many first-rate doctors out of the system and making the practice of medicine far less humane.

America pays more money per capita for health care than any other country in the world, yet millions of Americans have no health care coverage at all. Millions more have partial coverage.

Anyone who's ever had cancer clings to her job, quite literally, for dear life, knowing she may never get insurance again. Every American knows that if he's thrown out of work, if his company's health care plan changes or becomes balky, then he's only one serious illness away from penury. It's a truth to which thousands of people currently living in cars and on the streets can attest. Poor people in this country die of cancer much faster than people in the middle class.

Yet try telling Americans that this kind of suffering isn't tolerated in most industrialized countries. That just over the border, in Canada, there's a compassionate system, where patients are allowed free choice of doctors and hospitals, and where medical care is available to everyone. I have talked to Canadians who marvel at stories like Molly's. "I needed a bone marrow transplant," said one, "so I just presented my card at the hospital. I can't imagine having to fight for the money at the same time I'm fighting for my life. It just seems too cruel."

But American politicians simply dismiss the possibility of a Canadian-style system. They prefer to balance the budget by what they call "managed care." They win public support for this concept by talking about the horrendous amount of money currently spent on painful, futile treatments in the last days of the average patient's life. But managed care doesn't just mean withholding useless treatments. It means depriving people of medical care that might help or even cure them. In Oregon, for example, a plan has been proposed (implementation was prevented by George Bush) that would expand coverage for poor people, while denying them hundreds of specific treatments. If a cancer patient were judged terminal, this plan would withhold treatment. Yet treatment can often add years of productive life—occasionally even a normal lifespan. My friend Sara Wolfe was told many years ago that she had less than a 5 percent chance of surviving her cancer. She's now the healthy mother of two beautiful infants. Under the Oregon plan—which is being studied as a model by health care experts around the country—she would be dead.

Our pundits insist that a Canadian-style system is not economically feasible. Yet we currently waste around 20 percent of our health care dollar on paperwork. The insurance companies siphon off profits, while adding nothing to the system. How does it control costs to add a thick layer of bureaucrats to micromanage every relationship between doctor and patient?

There may be some limits to the health care that Americans have a right to expect, but before sick and desperate people are denied help, policymakers might consider limiting the runaway profits of drug companies, hospitals, doctors and particularly insurance companies.

If the stakes weren't so high, the contention that Canada's spending is out of control would be laughable. The U.S. system is such a mess of competing payers, Gordian knots of paperwork and mindless regulation that not one of the experts who so knowledgeably pontificate on health care really knows exactly what it costs. In Canada, with its far simpler system, every penny is tracked.

Our environmental crisis can't be solved by telling Americans to recycle plastic forks, nor can cancer be cured through meditation and vegetarianism. Individual empowerment is a fine thing, but it is only a beginning.

Cancer patients must come together with those who love us and those at risk for the disease—which is everyone in the country. We must use the clarity and compassion we've so painfully acquired to find the cause of the epidemic and agitate for a cure. We must make it our concern that every man, woman and child receive the best, the most loving and healing, care possible. We must take our mutilated bodies and our bald heads, our tears and our anger out into the streets and tell the others. First comes a time for introspection. Then comes the time to act.

APPENDIX B
WHAT I WISH I'D KNOWN
WHEN I WAS FIRST DIAGNOSED

The news that you have cancer may come soon after a biopsy or a few days later in a consultation with your doctor or on the phone. However it comes, it tends to leave you stunned and terrified. I asked several long-term breast cancer survivors what they know now that they wish they'd known at that moment.

They mentioned facts ranging from the practical and immediate through the emotional and spiritual. Here's a brief summary of their thoughts.

Time. Your panic at the diagnosis may be enhanced by the belief that you need to make immediate decisions about surgery. Your doctor may also insist on this. Be aware that most experts think you can safely give yourself a couple of weeks' breathing space before making a decision.

Information. For all of us, the diagnosis started a frantic search for information: We had only a week or two in which to decide between lumpectomy and mastectomy, not much longer to think about chemotherapy. "I wish I'd known where to turn for a comprehensive overview," said one friend who has survived her cancer by ten years. "I wanted a number or a person that could give me all the relevant facts about my particular cancer in a form I could digest and deal with."

Though I don't believe such a number exists, the Physicians' Data Query, listed in the resource guide (appendix C), gives up-to-date information and a list of experimental protocols. Many of the major research institutions have information lines, too. There are also some excellent books (see resource guide). Support organizations like QuaLife maintain libraries, and your local branch of the American Cancer Society can be very helpful. Your doctor should be able to direct you to a support organization.

Your doctor. I wish I'd been more resistant to the blanket condemnations of the medical profession that critics and feminists (myself among them) tended to make. I also wish I'd understood that the spurt of sheer hatred I felt toward my surgeon in the beginning was irrational. I've since learned that patients often leave the doctor who first tells them they have cancer. My doctors turned out to be caring people, up on the latest research and dedicated to healing.

I'd also question the almost universal recommendation to take the decision-making process into your own hands—at least in one respect. It's fine to prowl medical libraries and talk to everyone you've ever known who might have a smidgen of useful information, but you cannot find out enough to save your own life in two or three frantic weeks of searching. And if you try, you will hear enough sense and nonsense mixed to leave you reeling.

What you must take into your own hands is selection of a doctor. If you and your doctor don't communicate well, if she or he does not seem to be keeping abreast of developments in the field, by all means go doctor-shopping. I have friends who traveled throughout the country in search of experts, both conventional and alternative, though few patients have the emotional stamina or the money for this, and women with children would probably find it impossible.

Locally, you can ask a friend with good connections in the medical community for advice. Don't just ask another patient. Patients are as apt to feel irrational love for their doctors as irrational hatred. If there is nobody first-rate in your town, go to a major cancer center. Your doctor or librarian can help you find one.

How do you know if your doctor is competent? Look for a surgeon who specializes in breast cancer or who is known to do a number of such surgeries.

Although there are cases where mastectomy is necessary, expect your surgeon to prefer lumpectomy and to give good reasons if he recommends breast removal. You might also find out which he does most often. In most cases, lumpectomy is as good as mastectomy, and up-to-date surgeons are well aware of this.

Your oncologist should be able to give you convincing reasons and cite supporting statistics for whatever protocol she recommends. When you ask about something you've read in the newspaper or have heard from a friend, she should be aware of the study or trend you're talking about and able to discuss it knowledgeably.

Take a calm friend or a tape recorder, or both, to every session with your doctor as a reality check. I've never known any doctor to be offended by this. If yours is, dump him. Most doctors know that patients can't hear much that they're told in the first frightening weeks after diagnosis.

Other patients. Medical knowledge is best culled from professional journals, competent secondary sources and your doctor. But a different, and nourishing, kind of information comes from other cancer patients. One friend, mentioning this, added emphatically that she's not talking about "the cheerful types who bounce their exercise balls into your hospital room after your mastectomy to teach you arm exercises," but people who will acknowledge your fear and confusion and share their own.

Other patients will also tell you things your doctor might not think to or doesn't know. "I wanted to know what it felt like when they opened a vein and poured in the chemo," said my friend. "Not from someone doing it, but from someone it was done to."

You may not feel like calling a woman you've heard has survived breast cancer or joining a support group right away. It may seem weak or silly, or too much of an acknowledgment that your cancer is real. But I can't tell you what a pleasure it was when I first sat down with other cancer patients and heard my own fears, furies and joys coming from their lips. You can be completely honest with these companions. The feelings you keep from your loved ones for fear of burdening them spring loose; you are able to speak of death; you can make spiteful comments about those who are still healthy; you can make stupid cancer jokes. I'd leave some of these sessions almost dizzy with relief.

It's possible that the leader of the first support group you find will insist on maintaining a tone of relentless optimism, delivering endless exhortations to drink carrot juice and "keep a smile on your face." Or the overall tone may be unrelentingly gloomy. Unless you find these approaches helpful, search for another group, or pin a notice to your doctor's bulletin board and at least arrange to meet other patients.

Living with uncertainty. No matter how indefatigable your search, you will never find one incontrovertible truth about your cancer and its cure, just theories and hypotheses. You'll discover that the expert at Stanford disagrees with the expert at Sloan-Kettering. For a few months, every time you hear of someone who's chosen a different treatment from yours, you may feel threatened.

You need to know that this is the most difficult part of the entire process. Once you've decided on a course of action, you'll become much calmer. At that point, stop researching and vacillating and cultivate faith in your doctor and your treatment decisions.

Cancer politics. There are people who say that surgery causes cancer to spread and chemotherapy weakens the immune system, which would otherwise be able to destroy tumor cells. They argue that conventional approaches should be altogether avoided and recommend clinics and centers around the country that provide alternative therapies (see "Alternative Approaches" in the resource guide).

There's enough truth to these arguments to make them seductive. In the last few years, however, I have met or heard of several people who refused all standard treatments in favor of these alternative modes. By and large, they have not done well. Surgery, radiation and chemotherapy are limited and crude devices, but—despite all the propaganda to the contrary—they do have some good effect. Last year I read a study that showed that patients with several kinds of cancer actually lived longer in the United States, with its very aggressive modes of treatment, than patients with the same cancers elsewhere in the industrialized world.

However, I believe strongly in using alternative therapies in conjunction with standard treatments or when the benefits of standard treatments are dubious. Eating well, visualization, carrot juice, vitamins—I believe all these are helpful, and they enhance your sense of control. I still see a Chinese doctor regularly. Another friend, who has survived a brain metastasis by several years, swears by extract of mistletoe. (You can find it in *Third Opinion*, listed in the resource guide.) I'd advise an open, thoughtfully skeptical attitude toward tales of miraculous cure and some careful research.

Surgery. I wish I'd known that lumpectomy, node dissection and even mastectomy are generally not very painful or dangerous surgeries. But I also wish I'd understood how emotionally devastating any kind of cancer surgery is, how upsetting I'd find the thick tube dangling from my armpit for over a week after the node dissection, how long it would take me to fully accept my body again after such a betrayal.

On a practical level, I wish I'd known about studies showing that the timing of breast cancer surgery is very important. Premenopausal women seem to survive much longer if their tumors are removed during the second half of their monthly cycles. This is still contested in some medical circles, but the figures are quite dramatic. It can't hurt to schedule your surgery for twelve to sixteen days after your last menstrual period. Do the same for any biopsy.

Chemotherapy. I wish I'd known that the odd moments of forgetfulness I suffered were caused by the drugs and were not an incipient brain tumor, that confusion and depression were primarily side effects and would pass when the chemotherapy was over.

The protocol I was given left me able to work, though I was increasingly tired and cranky as time went on. Some people have more difficult reactions; some chemotherapies are more devastating. Don't try to measure yourself against someone else. If you're tired, rest; if you're unhappy, complain; if you want to spend the evenings snuggled on the sofa watching funny videos, do it; if salami sandwiches and a bar of chocolate make you feel less sick, indulge. You can clean up your diet later. The fact that your neighbor can jog three miles the day after her injection and you can't doesn't mean she's a better person or has a better prognosis.

Be kind to yourself—during treatment and for the entire first year or two.

Also: Be aware that, no matter how lacking in vanity you generally are, you're almost certain to be devastated when your hair falls out. It's normal. It passes. It helps if you've selected an attractive turban or wig beforehand.

The end of treatment. Although you've longed for this time, you may find yourself depressed when your treatments are over. You've been deserted by all the comforting people in white and left alone to face your fears. Plan time with your family or some specially supportive friends.

Happiness. It's good to know eventually you'll find yourself laughing, playing and actively involved in the world again. In the middle of my chemo treatments, I had lunch with an old friend who was complaining bitterly about her life. Words of comfort didn't seem to help. Suddenly I thought with wonder, "I'm happier than she is. Much happier. And I have cancer."

Several of the friends I asked said they wish they'd known sooner how mind steadying meditation could be. "It helps me just focus on the moment," said one. "Afterwards, I tell myself, I'm getting up from my chair ... I see the pattern on the carpet ... I open the refrigerator ... And right here, in the moment, I'm absolutely safe."

I would also like to have known what a powerful support system I had in my family, friends and co-workers and how true that corny old sixties anthem was that said, "Love is all you need."

Guilt. It would have saved a lot of anguish if I'd really understood what nonsense all the theories about the cancer personality are and how much pain they give to patients. It's good to create a healthful lifestyle and to try and keep your mind steady, but it's just plain stupid to believe that some personal deficiency or bad habit of thinking caused your cancer. I've met many unpleasant, negative people in the last few years who have survived their cancers and many beautiful, joyous souls who have succumbed. No matter how relentless the proselytizers of this theory may be—and they are everywhere—understand that it has not been proven and is highly suspect. Don't listen to anyone who implies you're in any way at fault for getting sick.

Statistics. Your doctor will say they're only a general guide and far from infallible, but you'll still seize on every figure that seems hopeful and freak out whenever a number sounds threatening. My oncologist says he's known women with tiny, noninvasive tumors who have done badly, others with dozens of affected lymph nodes who have survived for decades. There's no way of puzzling it out. Learn to treasure every day; learn to rest in the riddle.

Living with fear. There is no "over" with cancer. Your friends and family, satisfied that you're fine, may eventually go back about their business, but you'll still be worried every time you have a sore throat or a vague ache, still have nightmares when you have to go in for tests. Living with the full understanding that you're mortal is very difficult; in some ways it's also very rewarding.

My friends had a final piece of advice. Be sure and write down, they directed me, that we all wish we'd known, when we first heard that terrible word *cancer*, how rich and satisfying our lives could be so many years down the road.

APPENDIX C
RESOURCE GUIDE

Here's an idiosyncratic and highly selective list of resources that I found particularly helpful.

Books in General

Breast Cancer: The Complete Guide, by Yashar Hirshaut, M.D., and Peter I. Pressman, M.D. Bantam, 1992, $24.50.

Dr. Susan Love's Breast Book, by Susan M. Love with Karen Lindsey. Addison Wesley, 1991, $14.95. Kind, wise, comprehensive, a doctor's book brimming with necessary information.

Women Talk About Breast Surgery, by Amy Gross and Dee Ito. HarperCollins, 1991, $10.95. Oral accounts by patients.

The Women's Cancer Book, by Carolyn Faulder. Virago Press, Ltd., 20–23 Mandela Street, Camden Town, London NW1, England, 1989, 5 pounds, 99 pence. Calm, thoughtful and, since it's by an Englishwoman, providing a slightly different perspective.

The Web That Has No Weaver: Understanding Chinese Medicine, by Ted J. Kaptchuk. Congdon and Weed, 1983, $14.95.

The New Our Bodies, Ourselves, the Boston Women's Health Book Collective. Simon and Schuster's Touchstone Books, 1992, $20.00.

The Breast Cancer Companion: From Diagnosis to Recovery: Everything You Need to Know for Every Step Along the Way, by Kathy LaTour. Morrow, 1993, $22.00

The Magic Bullet

Natural Obsessions: The Search for the Oncogene, by Natalie Angier. Warner Books, 1989, $14.95. An incisive, elegantly written account of the way biomedical science is conducted that's as absorbing as fiction.

Cell Wars: The Immune System's Newest Weapons Against Cancer, by Marshall Goldberg, M.D. Fromm International Publishing Corporation, 1989, $8.95. A lively, intelligent account of work on monoclonal antibodies that gives an idea of what bioengineering is all about. Most important, it fills the reader with hope.

The Body Victorious, by Lennart Nilsson. Delacorte Press, 1987, $25.00. Magnificent color photos of the immune system in action.

Conceptualizing Illness

Love, Medicine and Miracles: Lessons Learned About Self-Healing from a Surgeon's Experience with Exceptional Patients, by Bernie S. Siegel, M.D. HarperCollins, 1990, $12.00. I have my disagreements with Siegel, but this is a warm and compassionate book.

Head First: The Biology of Hope, by Norman Cousins. Thorndike Press, 1991, $13.95. An intelligent exploration of the mind–body connection.

Illness as Metaphor and AIDS and Its Metaphors, by Susan Sontag. Doubleday, 1990, $8.95. A bracing debunking of prevalent myths.

Any book by physician-writer Richard Selzer.

Alternative Approaches

Third Opinion: An International Directory to Alternative Therapy Centers for the Treatment and Prevention of Cancer and Other Degenerative Diseases, by John M. Fink. Avery Publishing Group, 1992, $14.95.

Unconventional Cancer Treatments, a Congressional report available from the Superintendent of Documents, U.S. Government Printing Office, Washington, DC 20402–9325, 1990, $14.00. There has been some controversy about this document, with critics charging that the alternative therapies it reviews were given too short shrift. Still, an interesting document.

Michael Lerner of Commonweal, P.O. Box 316, Bolinas, CA 94924, (415) 868–0970, remains one of the country's top experts on alternative treatments. The organization provides information.

The Cancer Survivors and How They Did It, by Judith Glassman. Doubleday, 1983, $18.95. Glassman interviews patients who survived against all odds. Some used conventional methods, and some unconventional; Glassman searches for a common thread.

Diet and Lifestyle

Your Defense Against Cancer: The Complete Guide to Cancer Prevention, by Henry Dreher. Harper & Row, 1988, $19.95. A good overview of current opinions about diet, personality and lifestyle. This book appears to be out of print but should be available in libraries or used book stores.

Formula for Life: The Definitive Book on Correct Nutrition, Anti-Oxidants and Vitamins, Disease Prevention and Longevity, by Eberhard and Phyllis Kronhausen and Harry B. Demopoulos,

M.D. William Morrow, 1990, $14.95. Prepare to give up mushrooms, potato skins and alfalfa sprouts along with fats, salt and sugar if you find these authors convincing.

Vitamins in Cancer Prevention and Treatment: A Practical Guide, by Kedar N. Prasad. Healing Arts Press, 1 Park Street, Rochester, VT 05767, 1994, $9.95. A researcher in the field, Prasad offers no panaceas, just a practical little book detailing what's currently known.

Sharing the Experience

Examining Myself: One Woman's Story of Breast Cancer Treatment and Recovery, by Musa Meyer. Faber and Faber, 1993, $19.95.

Cancer Stories: Creativity and Self-Repair, by Esther Dreifuss-Kattan. The Analytic Press, Inc., 1990, $33.95. Although Dreifuss-Kattan's terminology and approach are a little foreign to me, this is my favorite among all the cancer books I've read. Quoting from writers as diverse as Tolstoy and Betty Rollins, she goes more deeply and beautifully into the psyche of those who are ill or dying than I'd ever imagined possible.

It's Always Something, by Gilda Radner. Avon Books, 1990, $5.95. A sad, funny, appealing book.

Cancer in Two Voices, by Sandra Butler and Barbara Rosenblum. Spinsters Book Company, 1991, $12.95. Rosenblum was a breast cancer patient, Butler her lover. The observations of these two intelligent women are worth hearing.

The Cancer Journals, by Audre Lorde. Aunt Lute, 1980, $7.00. Powerful and passionately feminist.

Her Soul Beneath the Bone: Women's Poetry on Breast Cancer, edited by Leatrice H. Lifshitz. University of Illinois Press, 1988, $10.95.

Spinning Straw into Gold: Your Emotional Recovery from Breast Cancer, by Ronnie Kaye. Simon and Schuster, 1991, $9.95. I'm not fond of self-help books, but this one is wise, kind and never simplistic.

One in Three: Women with Cancer Confront an Epidemic, edited by Judy Brady. Cleis Press, 1991, $10.95. The women whose essays are collected in this book deal with the politics of cancer, the medical profession, living with the disease and dying. They express emotions ranging from terror to joy, fury to love. My favorite is Anna Shaler's "Construction," a humorous, life-affirming tale of a one-breasted woman and the construction worker she takes to her bed. This book is also a good guide to cancer politics.

Tapes and Video

Emmett Miller's relaxation tapes can be obtained from Source, P.O. Box W, Stanford, CA 94309, or by calling 1–800–52TAPES.

Silence Like Glass, Media Home Entertainment, Inc., is a beautiful small film that was never generally released in this country. Jami Gertz stars as a young dancer who has cancer; Martha Plimpton is her dying roommate on the cancer ward. This is a bleak movie and difficult to watch, but ultimately I found it deeply healing. There wasn't a moment that struck me as false, and Gertz and Plimpton should receive Oscars for their fierce and lovely performances.

Organizations and Information

The Physicians' Data Query is a phone line run by the National Cancer Institute: 1–800–4–CANCER. It's used by doctors but is also available to the general public, and provides general information and an up-to-date list of all current experimental protocols.

The National Women's Health Network, 1325 G Street NW, Washington, DC 20005, (202) 347–1140. This group researches issues like the pill–breast cancer connection, the uses of tamoxifen, silicone gel in breast implants. Very efficient, very helpful.

Boston Women's Health Book Collective, Box 192, West Somerville, MA 02144. Publishers of *Our Bodies, Ourselves.*

National Coalition for Cancer Survivorship, 1010 Wayne Avenue, 5th floor, Silver Springs, MD 20910, (301) 650–8868. An advocacy group for cancer patients.

National Alliance of Breast Cancer Organizations, 2280 Avenue of the Americas, New York, NY 10036, (212) 719–0154. Publishes a newsletter that costs $25 a year.

Breast Cancer Coalition, P.O. Box 66373, Washington, DC 20035, (202) 296–7747. Does some good lobbying for increased research funds in Washington.

American Cancer Society, 1599 Clifton Road NE, Atlanta, GA 30329.

In Canada, the Cancer Information Service is a hotline for callers with questions about any type of cancer: 1–800–263–6750 (within Ontario); (416) 387–1153 (elsewhere in Canada). Its staffers will answer questions, provide statistics and direct people to various other services.

Order Form
for *Breast Cancer Journal*
by Juliet Wittman

Breast cancer is one of the most dire women's health issues of our time, striking one in *eight* American women. Any woman facing the disease—as well as family and friends of patients—will find strength in Juliet Wittman's *Breast Cancer Journal* because Juliet's book is not about breast cancer as cold statistics or clinical specimens; it's about a woman's life.

To order *Breast Cancer Journal* simply fill out this form and send to Fulcrum Publishing. Or order toll-free by calling **(800) 992-2908**.

Send ____ copies of *Breast Cancer Journal* at $14.95 each

Subtotal_____

Tax_____   Colorado residents add 4.3% tax

Shipping_____   Shipping: $3 for the first book, $1 for each additional book

TOTAL_____

❑ Check or money order enclosed (Make checks payable to Fulcrum Publishing.)

Please charge my:
❑ VISA   ❑ MasterCard   ❑ American Express

Card #_____Expiration Date_____

Signature_____

❑ Check here to receive our catalog of books and calendars

Send orders to:
Fulcrum Publishing
350 Indiana St., Suite 350
Golden, CO
80401-5093
800-992-2908

SHIP TO:

Name_____

Address_____

City_____State_____ Zip_____

Phone_____